Differential Diagnosis

Differential Diagnosis

A guide to symptoms and signs of
common diseases and disorders,
presented in systematic form

Alexander D. G. Gunn

MRCGP, DObstRCOG, DPH
Director, University Health Services
University of Reading
United Kingdom

SP MEDICAL & SCIENTIFIC BOOKS

New York

Published in the UK by
MTP Press Limited
Falcon House
Lancaster
England

SPECTRUM PUBLICATIONS, INC.
175-20 Wexford Terrace, Jamaica, N.Y. 11432

ISBN 0-89335-159-8

Library of Congress Catalogue Card No. 81-52913

Contents

List of Differential Diagnosis Tables

Foreword

This book is designed for use by medical students, nurses, young practitioners, internists, family physicians and all those initially involved with the problem of diagnostics. It is structured to provide a concise logical approach to the diagnosis of common illness and disorders in adults. The elucidation of an illness cause is not easy for the inexperienced. Although textbooks and guidance notes can be referred to for clarification of assembled thought – once a medical history has been taken – a system-orientated reference guide has considerable value for aiding and checking the logic of diagnosis.

It is hoped that this book will fulfil that purpose. It could not have been written without the help of R. G. Brackenridge's *Essential Medicine* (1979, MTP, Lancaster, England), and J. Fry's *Common Diseases* (1979, MTP, Lancaster, England), to which the reader is referred and to which generous acknowledgement is made. The tables of Differential Diagnosis that follow Chapters 3–7 are adapted from some that have appeared in *Handbook of Differential Diagnosis*, vols 1–3, published by Rocom Press, Hoffman La Roche Inc., New Jersey, 1968–1974 – an invaluable publication now unfortunately out of print, and permission to do so is gratefully appreciated. Finally without the stimulus and encouragement of Mr David Bloomer (MTP) and the particular assistance of Mrs J. C. Robinson, this book would never have been written.

ALEXANDER D. G. GUNN

Reading, Berks, UK
1981

Chapter 1

Introduction – How to Use this Book for Reference

A guide to differential diagnosis, unless it ran to several volumes, could never encompass all aspects of every known form of disorder or disease. The common disorders and illnesses, however, wherever they are met, share the specific characteristics of common symptoms and signs that can be elicited in taking the patient's history and in the physical examination that follows. In general an illness will affect one or other of the patient's major physical systems and this book provides reference systematically to the common disorders and illnesses – by listing the symptoms and signs and describing the routine diagnostic investigations. As a revision course in preparing for examinations, the major differential aspects of diagnoses are listed in the text and tabled at the end of the relevant chapters. As a guide to the key laboratory investigations in diagnosis, the chapters and the tables detail the routines that would apply in confirming the suspicion formed by examination of the patient. No book, however, will ever replace the wisdom gained by experience in the practice of medicine and all practitioners will need to constantly update their knowledge of medical science by continued reading of the relevant literature. This book, therefore, is a guide, logically presenting information about illness and disorder that enables the doctors or students of medicine and nursing newly in practice to check and constantly improve their diagnostic ability.

When a patient's history has been taken, the first step in the clinical reasoning process is to decide which of the findings that have been elicited are relevant to the discovery of the possible disease. The initial symptoms are those which are presented by way of verbal communication; other symptoms are elicited and the signs of disorder are detected by the physical examination – but this has to be done in a routine manner in order to ask the specific cross-checking questions. Differential diagnosis is essentially a process of logical thought – not dissimilar from a mental flow chart as written for computer programming. Focusing on a system disorder enables the clinician to consider all the likely possible causes and to reflect on the necessary laboratory tests for ultimate confirmation. Sixty per cent of the diagnosis is made at the history-taking stage in the experienced – since the practice of medicine is essentially that of problem analysis. The patient presents with the problem, the clinician has to know, or define, its common causes, be aware of its more probable cause in that specific patient, and to ascertain through examination and laboratory testing the specific cause for that particular patient – in order to provide any form of therapeutic advice or management. It is a process of systematically testing hypotheses.

The first hypothesis, therefore, is the patient claiming that there is a system disorder. Each chapter of this book opens with a brief survey of the frequency of such system illnesses and their broadest epidemiological pattern. The diagnoses of common disorders, however, depend on certain particular types or forms of clinical investigation – be it blood test, urine examination, X-ray etc., and these are listed to act as an *aide memoire* for the clinician. The common relevant symptoms are then listed, to be followed by further discussion of the appropriate tests. Thus, before reaching the text detailing the disorders themselves, the reader is primed with the basis of problem-solving knowledge. The common disorders and diseases are then described and detailed, with causes and the specific symptoms and signs listed. Recommendations with regard to further investigations are made where appropriate. The pattern of the text, therefore, is that of initial broad consideration of the diseases, epidemiologically, followed by clinical and diagnostic detail.

Chapter 2
The Medical History

Taking a medical history is a skill, acquired by most as a result of experience and taught to the student as the very basis of all diagnostic accuracy. It is an interview that should be structured between patient and clinician and from it has to emerge:

(1) the reason the patient sought help,
(2) the circumstances and details of the illness,
(3) the previous medical history,
(4) a family history,
(5) an occupational history,
(6) medication taken, and current or previous attempts to modify or treat the symptoms,
(7) social drug usage (tobacco, alcohol or others),
(8) an assessment of the function of the main body systems.

Whilst the interview is taking place, the clinician will be forming a further assessment of two important factors relevant to the diagnosis:

(1) the severity of the complaint,
(2) its relevance to that individual's life pattern.

There are, however, only two questions that require answering with regard to the problem posed:

What is its cause?
What are its consequences?

In these two questions lie the whole direction of the clinician's subsequent activity, for they determine the process of the routine physical examination, the laboratory investigations, the confirmation of the diagnosis and the ultimate treatment and follow-up. Thus diagnosis is essentially the answering of these questions.

At the history-taking stage, these questions will be in the mind of the clinician from the very beginning – they are implicit even if the patient is unconscious and unable to verbally communicate at all. In the routine of the standard medical interview, however, they are constantly guiding the interrogative remarks and direction of both conversations. Although the patient cannot necessarily present the information to the doctor in the ideal logical form that answers them – the patient actually has the same questions in mind, and has had ever since a disturbance of function has been noticed. There is thus – except in the mentally disordered, precomatose, or very ill – an implicit agreement that the medical history-taking is leading to the answers being produced. Cooperation, therefore, is usual; the difference in the relationship is that the doctor guides the conversation.

Verbal communication is, however, liable in all circumstances to be fraught with distraction, digression, misunderstanding, or failure in comprehension – on the part of both participants – that is why in medicine it has to be a mental discipline. Computer diagnosis, by means of question and answer through a visual display unit's keyboard, can never replace the empathy, voice tonality or demeanour recognition that can be conveyed only by human contact. Factual histories may be more rapidly, or in some cases, conveniently elicited but diagnostic histories are not always, or even simply, a matter of fact, they require impressions to be formed, attitudes to be assessed and important emphases to be recognized that cannot be conveyed by specific Yes–No answers.

A medical history is 'taken' from a patient, not given,

offered or simply produced – it is a process of extraction and distillation. That is why each chapter that follows emphasizes repetitively that any diagnosis of disorder *will depend on symptoms, history, observation of the patient and examination* of a routine series of recommendations. For the history-taking is an inseparable part of the observation of the patient and in it lies the art of medical practice – the science is in the confirmation of the diagnosis.

Chapter 3
The Cardiovascular System

The commonest disorders of the cardiovascular system are hypertension, coronary artery disease, varicose veins, heart failure, and cardiac arrhythmias, phlebitis and peripheral artery disease in that order of frequency. Death will be caused most frequently through coronary artery disease and 51% of all deaths in Britain and the USA are from circulatory disease. Disorder of the cardiovascular system is predominantly a result of age.

Diagnosis of disorder will depend on symptoms, history, observation of the patient and examination of:

(A) pulse,
(B) blood pressure,
(C) heart sounds (auscultation),
(D) electrical tracing of the heart muscle activity (electrocardiogram).

(A chest X-ray and serum electrolyte measurements with other blood tests will also be necessary)

Common symptoms of generalized disorder will be:

(1) breathlessness (on exertion or lying flat),
(2) cyanosis (blue discoloration of face, lips and fingertips),
(3) oedema (ankle swelling),
(4) chest pain,
(5) headaches,
(6) palpitations,
(7) confusion or restlessness,
(8) loss of consciousness.

(A) EXAMINATION OF THE PULSE

Consider the rate, rhythm and force of the pulse. The normal rate is 60–80 per minute.

RATE

A rapid pulse, tachycardia, can result from increased metabolism (exercise, emotion, fevers, thyrotoxicosis), blood loss, and cardiac disorders.

A slow pulse, bradycardia, occurs in simple faint (syncope, vasovagal attack), heart block, and digoxin overdosage.

RHYTHM

Irregularity occurs in:

Sinus arrhythmia – normal in youth, the pulse rate increases with inspiration, and decreases on expiration.

Paroxysmal tachycardia – sudden burst of regular beating, rate 150–200; not usually a sign of heart disease, but heart failure may occur if the attack is prolonged.

Atrial fibrillation – due to:
(1) rheumatic heart disease involving the mitral valve,
(2) ischaemic (coronary) heart disease,
(3) thyrotoxicosis.

The atria are twitching rapidly and irregularly at around 300–400 'beats' per minute. The conducting bundle cannot respond to such a high rate, and the ventricles beat at an irregular 100–200 per minute.

Atrial flutter – this is relatively rare and may be caused by the same heart diseases as atrial fibrillation. The atrium is 'fluttering' at a regular 200–400 beats per minute, again there is a block (which may be variable) in the conducting tissues, and the ventricular rate is less than 150, generally regular.

Extrasystoles (ectopic beats) – these arise from an abnormal focus in the atria (supraventricular extrasystoles) or in the ventricles. They may be unimportant, with no associated heart disease, or important in digoxin poisoning (coupled beats) and after myocardial infarction.

Heart block – due to some or all of the stimuli from the atrial pacemaker failing to reach the ventricular muscle. Thus the block may be incomplete with missed beats and irregular rhythm, or complete when the ventricle takes up its own rhythm at a regular 40 beats per minute or less. Heart block may occur in myocardial infarction.

(B) EXAMINATION OF THE BLOOD PRESSURE

The blood pressure is measured with the sphygmomanometer. The cuff is applied to the upper arm, inflated until the mercury is above the level where the pulse is no longer palpable, then deflated while one listens with the stethoscope over the brachial artery. The level at which pulse sounds become audible is called the systolic blood pressure. As the cuff is deflated further, the sounds become faint and then inaudible. This is the diastolic reading. The systolic pressure depends on the force of the cardiac contraction and the state of the walls of the large vessels, being higher in the elderly whose vessels are harder and less elastic than those in young people. The diastolic pressure corresponds to the resting pressure in the artery between heart beats. The intensity of the blood pressure sounds may be diminished if the cardiac output is poor, when it may be difficult to be sure of the systolic and diastolic readings, and it is not always possible to record within 2 mm. A fat arm causes a falsely high reading. The normal blood pressure is:

$$\frac{100\text{–}140 \text{ (systolic)}}{70\text{–}90 \text{ (diastolic)}}$$

A falling blood pressure indicates haemorrhage or deteriorating cardiac function, but cardiac disease may exist with a normal blood pressure.

(C) EXAMINATION OF THE HEART SOUNDS

The heart is a muscular pump with four chambers – the right atrium, which receives venous blood from the systemic veins; the right ventricle, which pumps the blood through the pulmonary artery to the lungs to be oxygenated; the left atrium, which receives this blood from the lungs; and the left ventricle, which pumps blood through the aorta to reach arteries and capillaries throughout the body.

At each beat the ventricles contract simultaneously to expel their blood, the heart valves (tricuspid and pulmonary on the right side, mitral and aortic valves on the left) preventing backward flow. The heart beat causes a wave palpable as the pulse in a peripheral artery. The heart sounds, audible with the stethoscope over the 'apex' medial to the left nipple, are two in number, 'lup–dup'. They are due to the valves closing at the beginning and end of the contraction phase, which is called systole, and this is followed by the resting and filling phase, or diastole.

(D) ELECTROCARDIOGRAM

Cardiac contraction is 'fired' by an electrical stimulus, arising at the pacemaker in the sinoatrial node, spreading through the right atrium to reach the atrioventricular node, then down an electrical 'bundle' between the ventricles; this bundle divides into two branches and the stimulus thence passes out into the ventricular muscle (myocardium). This tiny electric current can be detected by applying plates or 'electrodes' to the chest and limbs, and recorded on paper or displayed on an oscilloscope (monitor) – the electrocardiogram (ECG).

Disturbances of rate and rhythm may arise anywhere in the electrical conducting system. While they may be detectable by feeling the pulse or by listening to the heart, an ECG is essential for accurate diagnosis and treatment.

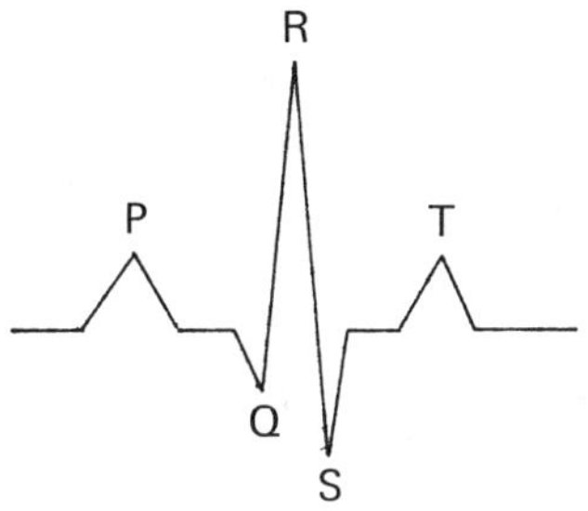

The P wave denotes atrial activity, the QRS complex and the T wave ventricular activity.

Common Disorders of the Cardiovascular System

(1) HYPERTENSION (HIGH BLOOD PRESSURE)

The normal blood pressure ranges from 120/80 for a person in his twenties to about 160/90 in his sixties. The diastolic level is raised from narrowing of small arteries and arterioles. A raised diastolic pressure is usually accompanied by a raised systolic pressure. The effects of hypertension on the heart, kidneys and retinae of the eyes are more important than arbitrary blood pressure readings, which may be influenced by emotion. The finding of a raised blood pressure in a symptomless patient should direct attention to these organs, and treatment will prevent further damage to them.

Rare causes

Coarctation of the aorta – a congenital narrowing of the aorta just beyond its origin at the heart; occurs in the young; radial pulses normal, but femoral pulses diminished or absent.

Adrenal gland causes.

Tumour of medulla, producing adrenaline-like substances excreted in the urine, causes hypertension, often paroxysmal, accompanied by sweating.

Over-activity of adrenal cortex, producing trunk obesity and skin 'staining' from excess cortisol production, measurable in the urine.

Tumour of adrenal cortex, producing polyuria, weakness and low serum potassium.

Common causes

Renal disease: chronic glomerulonephritis,
chronic pyelonephritis,
renal artery stenosis.

These may cause the kidney to produce renin, a substance which raises the blood pressure, and which also stimulates the adrenals to produce aldosterone, further raising the blood pressure.

Toxaemia of pregnancy – placental hormones may play a part, and there is accompanying albuminuria and oedema, and fits (eclampsia) in severe cases.

No definite cause can be found in the vast majority of cases, when the term essential hypertension is used. There may be a family history, suggesting a hereditary basis in some cases.

Symptoms and signs

The finding of a raised blood pressure is common, especially in women after the menopause; the condition may be symptomless and in the elderly it is often harmless. The symptoms and signs of hypertension are in fact due to its effects on the heart and blood vessels, especially the cerebral arteries and smaller vessels in the retina of the eye, and effects on the kidneys.

Headache is not a common complaint except in severe hypertension.

Epistaxis (nose bleeding) may be a mode of presentation.

Breathlessness. The left ventricle must pump against the increased pressure in the arteries, gradually enlarges, shows signs of strain detectable on ECG and eventually fails; the resultant pulmonary oedema causes breathlessness on exertion, and on lying flat in bed nocturnal dyspnoea.

Pre-existing coronary artery disease may be made worse.

Cerebral haemorrhage. Arteriosclerotic disease affecting the internal carotid artery and the intracerebral vessels is worsened and a vessel may break down causing cerebral haemorrhage (and often death); there is also an increased risk of cerebral thrombosis. The smaller intracranial arteries may be affected causing cerebral oedema, and the condition of hypertensive encephalopathy, with headaches, fits, disturbance of consciousness and transient episodes of paralysis.

Visual disturbance. The retinal arteries may be affected and severe cases have visual upset and retinal haemorrhages and papilloedema (blurring of the optic discs) – visible with the opthalmoscope.

Polyuria. Not only may kidney disease cause hypertension, but hypertension from any cause will in turn damage the kidneys. The renal units (nephrons) are gradually destroyed, and remaining nephrons work at maximum level, but the kidneys are no longer able to reproduce concentrated urine. They can only eliminate the body's waste products, such as urea, in large quantities of dilute urine (polyuria). The patient may admit to having to rise at night to pass urine, and may complain of thirst. The blood urea gradually rises, and if the condition is untreated, the patient passes into renal failure with dehydration, vomiting, coma and death.

These effects of hypertension may be very gradual, with progressive deterioration over many years. In some younger patients, however, the process is much more rapid, and is called malignant or accelerated hypertension – with very high diastolic pressure (over 140 mmHg), retinal haemorrhages and papilloedema, and progressive renal failure.

Investigations in hypertension

(1) Charting of the blood pressure.
(2) Urine: specific gravity – fixed at 10.10 with renal involve-

ment, may contain albumin; laboratory examination may show red cells and casts, and superadded renal infection causes pus cells and positive bacteriological culture (colony count); 24-hour specimens sent for corticosteroid assay (in suspected Cushing's syndrome).

(3) ECG – shows left ventricular enlargement or strain.
(4) Chest X-ray – shows enlarged heart, and early pulmonary oedema.
(5) Intravenous pyelogram X-ray (IVP) – assesses size and function of kidneys.
(6) Serum 'electrolytes' (sodium and potassium) and the blood urea level.

(2) CORONARY ARTERY DISEASE

Coronary heart disease is the commonest single cause of death amongst middle-aged men.

The heart muscle receives its blood supply from the coronary arteries, and these are affected with ageing, by the process of arteriosclerosis. Plaques of fatty material are laid down in the arterial lining (atheroma); calcium may be deposited in the plaques. Minute clots (thrombi) tend to form on the irregular surface, further narrowing the lumen (bore) of the artery so that the heart receives insufficient blood for its own needs.

Causes

High animal fat intake has been blamed, and also a diet too rich in refined carbohydrate and sugar. Arteriosclerosis is less common in races with a more natural diet including bran and fibre, and in those taking polyunsaturated oils rather than animal fats. A disturbance of the blood clotting mechanism has also been postulated.

Coronary heart disease is much commoner in men, but women who take oestrogen-containing contraceptive pills are at increased risk.

There is a definite association with heavy cigarette-smoking. Lack of exercise may also play a part. The stress and strains of modern life may have some effect as adrenaline release affects the blood fats. Raised blood pressure and obesity aggravate the condition.

Symptoms and signs

Angina pectoris

The blood supply through the narrowed coronaries is inadequate during effort; the impaired metabolism results in the formation of substances that cause pain.

There is a constricting central chest pain brought on by exercise, especially hill-climbing, or emotional excitement, and relieved by rest. The pain may radiate to the arms, especially the left arm, and the lower jaw. The patient may describe the tight feeling as one of difficulty in getting his breath. There are no consistent pulse or blood pressure changes, but patients generally have an abnormal ECG.

Myocardial infarction (heart attack)

This is due to a sudden blockage of a narrowed artery by clot, hence the term coronary thrombosis.

A part of the heart's blood supply is suddenly cut off, causing 'infarction' which means death of an area of tissue. If a vital part of the electrical conducting tissue is involved, even a small infarct may cause arrhythmia and sudden death from cardiac arrest (see below) yet the rest of the heart muscle may be undamaged. The infarct goes through processes of healing similar to those in a wound, scar tissue ultimately replacing the damaged area of myocardium.

There is chest pain, similar in site and distribution to angina, but more severe and prolonged, and not necessarily related to exertion – symptoms may arise when the patient is in bed. Severe pain is accompanied by sweating, nausea and vomiting, and by restlessness. There may be a feeling of extreme breathlessness and of impending doom.

Severe cases have pallor, cyanosis with cold extremities, irregularities of the pulse (which may be rapid or slow) hypotension, and rapidly developing pulmonary oedema and congestive heart failure.

Cardiac arrest

Cardiac arrest is due to ventricular fibrillation (the ventricular muscle twitching but failing to give a proper contraction) or to all its movements ceasing. In both cases there is a sudden failure of the circulation, and the brain can survive for only 3–4 min. It may have occurred through:

(1) myocardial infarction;
(2) pulmonary embolism, when the pulmonary circulation is blocked by clots from the veins;
(3) severe haemorrhage;
(4) electrocution and drowning.

There is sudden collapse, loss of consciousness, absence of pulse and of heart beat, increasing cyanosis often with gasping respiratory efforts; pupils become dilated and patient will die if left untreated.

Summon help – alarm call in hospital.

Lay patient flat on a firm surface (bed boards or the floor) but elevate the legs.

Give a sharp thump on the patient's chest – this may restart the heart. If not, proceed with external cardiac massage – apply the heel of one hand to the lower sternum and with the other hand on top compress the sternum backwards some 3–4 cm about 80 times per minute.

Artificial ventilation – remove false teeth, clear the airway by supporting the chin well forward, insert airway if available. Inflate the lungs by mouth-to-mouth breathing once for every five chest compressions.

Investigations in coronary artery diseases

(1) charting of blood pressure and pulse rate;
(2) charting of urine output;
(3) ECG and continual ECG monitoring;
(4) blood level assessment of cardiac muscle enzymes (SGOT and SLDH) and serum electrolytes;
(5) white cell count and ESR;
(6) chest X-ray – coronary angiogram (only in cases going on for cardiac surgery).

(3) HEART FAILURE

This may occur acutely, after massive myocardial infarction, or can be a gradual process over months or years. Often the heart muscle has enlarged despite ischaemia, or in the attempt to maintain cardiac output with diseased valves, but ultimately the myocardium fails.

Thus heart failure is pump failure. It is associated with salt and water retention, related to impaired circulation to the kidneys. Salt retention causes water retention, and the result is an excessive blood volume, so that the circulation becomes overloaded, further embarrassing the heart.

Causes

Left ventricular failure results from ischaemic, hypertensive, and aortic or mitral valve disease, for in these conditions the brunt of the trouble is borne by the left ventricle. Symptoms result from back-pressure on the vessels in the lungs, causing pulmonary oedema.

Right ventricular failure follows left ventricular failure, but may occur first in some cases of mitral stenosis where there is constriction of the blood vessels in the lung producing right ventricular strain.

Chronic bronchitis and emphysema also throw a strain on the right side of the heart.

Right ventricular failure results in systemic congestion – raised venous pressure, swollen liver and peripheral oedema.

Precipitating factors: in patients with known heart disease, heart failure may be precipitated by a further myocardial infarction or an episode of arrhythmia.

Intercurrent infection, especially respiratory infection, and anaemia are non-cardiac precipitating factors.

Symptoms and signs

Breathlessness – (dyspnoea, difficulty in breathing) may be noted first on exertion or stair-climbing. In left ventricular failure and pulmonary oedema, breathlessness when the patient is woken from sleep is characteristic. This occurs from increased lung congestion when the patient lies flat, and is relieved by sitting up in bed. In heart failure generally, patients feel less dyspnoeic when propped up. Severe pulmonary oedema causes extreme breathlessness and the production of frothy red sputum.

Cyanosis – blue discoloration of lips, cheeks and fingertips from sluggish peripheral circulation and reduced oxygen content of the blood in the capillaries. The skin is usually cold, except in heart failure following pulmonary disease, when the extremities may be warm.

Oedema – fluid retention in tissues and in heart failure is gravitational; thus there is oedema (pitting with finger pressure) over the ankles and legs, or above the sacrum if the patient has been confined to bed. Swelling of the abdomen may be due to ascites, fluid exudation into the peritoneal cavity. In right heart failure the jugular venous pressure is raised and pulsation is visible in the neck. The liver may be tender and swollen.

Restlessness and confusion – due to cerebral anoxia; there may be Cheyne–Stokes breathing from affection of the respiratory centre in the brain. This is a form of periodic breathing – depression of the respiratory centre causes apnoea (no breathing) followed by carbon dioxide retention which stimulates the centre into causing deep sighing respirations.

Pulse rate – usually raised, and may be regular or irregular. The commonest irregularity is atrial fibrillation with a rapid ventricular rate. Not all the beats of the heart may be strong enough to reach the periphery so that the apical rate may be higher than the pulse rate – pulse deficit.

Blood pressure – may be normal, raised (e.g. in hypertensive failure) or low; a low blood pressure associated with cold, blue extremities indicates poor cardiac output and carries a bad prognosis.

Lack of appetite, nausea and vomiting – occur from congestion of the stomach, and impaired circulation to the large bowel causes constipation or occasionally diarrhoea.

Urinary output – may be lowered from poor circulation to the kidneys, and there may be albuminuria. Electrolyte disturbances (sodium and potassium) are part of the picture of cardiac failure. Not only is there sodium and water retention, but there is also potassium loss rendering the heart more irritable and liable to arrhythmias.

Venous thrombosis – in the legs, with risk of pulmonary embolism, may occur from circulatory slowing, and is an important complication of cardiac failure.

(4) PERICARDITIS

Pericarditis is inflammation of the pericardial sac covering the heart. Pericarditis may be 'dry', or there may be a pericardial effusion.

Causes

As a complication of rheumatic fever (part of the 'carditis' of severe cases), or of myocardial infarction, and in the late stages of renal failure.

Acute viral infection.

Rheumatoid arthritis and collagen diseases.

Myxoedema.

Spread of infection from lung or pleura.

Symptoms and signs

In rheumatic fever and myocardial infarction the symptoms are mainly those of the underlying condition, with more superficial chest pain and a pericardial 'friction rub' heard with the stethoscope.

In young adults, where Coxsackie virus infection may be a cause, associated symptoms such as cough, sore throat and muscular pain are present.

There is fever and retrosternal pain.

There is a friction rub and typical ECG changes of pericarditis, but the myocardium is not involved to any extent and the cardiac enzymes (SGOT and SLDH) are not raised.

Pericarditis with effusion – these prevent the proper pumping action of the heart, especially the right ventricle, causing right

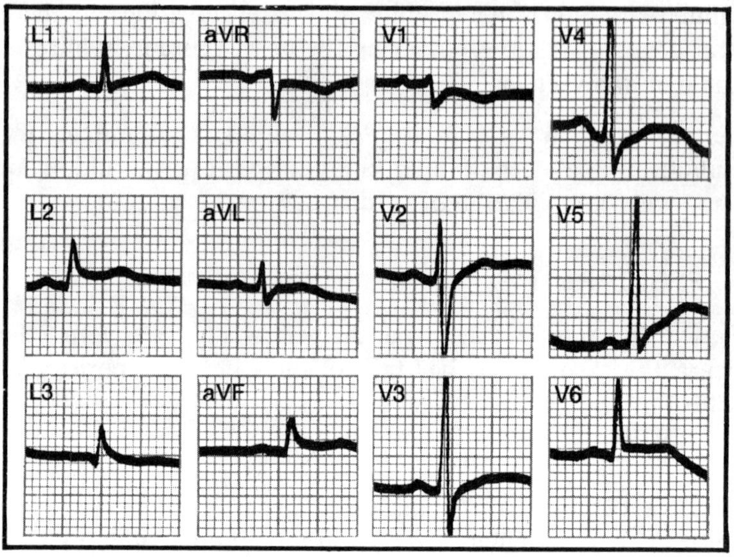

Electrocardiogram showing ST segment shifts appropriate to acute pericarditis

ventricular failure – distended neck veins, enlarged liver and peripheral oedema. These signs are out of proportion to breathlessness, and the patient may lie flat without dyspnoea as the lungs are not engorged.

There may be a complaint of weakness from poor cardiac output, with small pulse and low blood pressure.

In pericardial effusion the cardiac shadow on X-ray is enlarged.

Ultrasonic scanning may show fluid levels present.

(5) PULMONARY EMBOLISM

Causes

Arises from deep vein thrombosis in the leg.

Venous thrombosis is a complication of bed rest, especially in those with cardiac failure.

Obesity.

Following abdominal operations.

In those on the contraceptive 'pill'.

Symptoms and signs

In about half the cases there is evidence of leg vein thrombosis such as calf pain and oedema, but often the clot has arisen silently from upper parts of the vein in the thigh, and the first sign of trouble is in the lungs or heart:

Pulmonary infarction – pain on breathing, from pleural involvement.

Breathlessness.

Haemoptysis (blood in the sputum).

Rise in pulse rate.

A pleural rub may be heard with the stethoscope, and there may be X-ray changes.

Massive pulmonary embolus – a large clot may completely obstruct the pulmonary artery, with sudden collapse.

Severe breathlessness.

Cyanosis.

Chest pain.

Raised jugular venous pressure.

Rapid thready pulse with low or immeasurable blood pressure. Death will follow unless the clot breaks up or can be speedily removed surgically.

(Special investigations include pulmonary angiography and lung scanning with radioactive isotopes, but there may be no time for these in severe cases.)

(6) PERIPHERAL ARTERIAL AND VASCULAR DISEASE

The victims again are middle-aged men, and the elderly of both sexes. Cigarette-smoking and obesity are predisposing factors, and arteriosclerosis of the distal leg arteries, and those in the feet, is commoner in diabetics.

CHRONIC ARTERIOSCLEROSIS OF LOWER LIMB VESSELS

Cause

Arteriosclerotic narrowing and varying degrees of obstruction, involving the iliac arteries in the pelvis, and femoral vessels (and their branches) in the thigh. The condition may spread to involve distant arteries, but in diabetics vessels in the feet may be involved before there is gross disease.

Symptoms and signs

Intermittent claudication. The patient may complain that his pulses are impalpable, the leg loses its hairs, the skin is pale and may have a shiny appearance and is cool to the touch.

Wounds heal poorly and are liable to infection.

Severe cases develop 'rest pain,' occurring characteristically during the night, the patient putting his feet on a cold floor in an attempt to gain relief. This indicates extensive disease, with risk of skin breakdown and gangrene.

Investigations

Investigations should be made for conditions such as heart failure.

Anaemia.

Diabetes.

In younger patients in whom there is no evidence of generalized arterial disease, arteriography should be carried out to ascertain if there is a localized segment of arterial narrowing amenable to surgery.

ACUTE ARTERIAL OBSTRUCTION

Cause

This is usually an embolus from the left side of the heart, from thrombus in the left atrium in mitral stenosis, or from thrombus under a myocardial infarction. Clot may also become detached from a large arteriosclerotic vessel, or form over an existing arteriosclerotic plaque.

Symptoms and signs
Sudden severe pain.

Pallor (or cyanosis from associated venospasm).

Coldness.

Loss of sensation and muscular weakness in the affected limb.

Absent arterial pulses. Patients usually have a history of arterial disease, or may be in heart failure, but the condition may occur without previous symptoms.

RAYNAUD'S SYNDROME

This is due to spasm of the small arteries of the fingers and hands. It is commonest in young women, who complain of pallor and numbness of the fingers on exposure to cold.

Similar symptoms may occur in men using vibrating tools, and in autoimmune disorders such as scleroderma, where destruction of the small vessels, and gangrene, may follow.

VENOUS THROMBOSIS AND EMBOLISM

Deep vein thrombosis

This is the presence of thrombus (clot) in the deep veins of the calf, but the femoral vein in the thigh may also be involved.

Causes
Bed rest, especially if circulatory slowing occurs as in congestive cardiac failure.

Surgical operations; thrombus often develops at the time of operation, but spreads in the following days due to alterations in the coagulability of the blood.

Pregnancy, and contraceptive tablets of high oestrogen content. Neoplasm, often hidden, e.g., carcinoma of pancreas.

DIFFERENTIAL DIAGNOSIS OF CENTRAL CHEST PAIN

	Character	*Location*	*Radiation*	*Duration*
Angina pectoris	pressing crushing, bursting	substernal	shoulders, arms, neck, jaw	usually 1–3 min
Coronary insufficiency	pressing, crushing, bursting	substernal	shoulders, arms, neck, jaw	few minutes to several hours
Myocardial infarction	pressing crushing, bursting	substernal	shoulders, arms, neck, jaw	less than an hour to several days
Acute pericarditis	crushing or sharp	substernal	shoulders, neck, or back (not arms or jaws)	days to weeks
Pulmonary embolus	sudden and oppressive	substernal	chest, shoulders, epigastrium	minutes to hours; may recur

Onset	*Associated signs and symptoms*	*ECG changes*
exertion; emotional stress	fear and anxiety; patient pale, sometimes sweating; may have apical presystolic gallop rhythm to heart sounds	ECG may show ST depression during exercise
usually at rest	fear and anxiety; dyspnoea; patient pale and often sweating; may have fast pulse rate	ECG may show ST and T changes; temperature normal; SGOT elevation may be detected within first 7–14 days if infarct develops
usually at rest	fear and anxiety; dyspnoea; weakness; shock; arrhythmia; acute left ventricular failure	Q waves and other acute changes on ECG; SGOT and temperature elevated
usually at rest	fever; non-productive cough; pericardial friction rub; paradoxical pulse in more severe	ST elevation and T inversion in bipolar limb and precordial leads
usually at rest	marked dyspnoea; rapid shallow breathing, often cyanotic; low blood pressure; haemoptysis and pleural pain later	shift of QRS axis to right bundle branch block

Symptoms and signs

Calf pain and tenderness.

Ankle oedema.

Sometimes slight rise of temperature.

Investigations

Include the use of ultrasound with the portable Sonicaid detector, which fails to emit its characteristic flow-noise if the circulation is obstructed.

Injected radioactive fibrinogen may be detected at the site of thrombosis by using a special counter.

X-ray venography may be necessary to localize the site and extent accurately.

Superficial vein thrombosis (phlebitis)

Thrombosis in a superficial vein may occur after injury or use of indwelling cannulae for intravenous infusions. The condition may occur spontaneously in the legs, especially in relation to varicose veins.

Symptoms and signs

Local pain.

A red tender area along the line of the vein, which may be palpable as a thrombus-containing cord.

Chapter 4
The Respiratory System

Respiratory diseases are the most common cause of illness, at all ages, but account for a relatively small proportion of all hospital admissions. Acute respiratory infections and asthma are the most frequent cause of hospitalization in the younger patient, with chronic bronchitis, cancer of the lung and broncho-pneumonia in the older. Twenty per cent of all deaths in Britain and the USA are from respiratory disease, but with advancing age it is from pneumonia, chronic chest disease and lung cancer in that order of frequency.

Diagnosis of disorder will depend on symptoms, history of the patient and examination of:

(A) respiration rate and character,
(B) chest sounds (auscultation),
(C) chest X-ray,
(D) sputum,
(E) peak expiratory flow rate,
(F) blood gas analysis.

Common symptoms of respiratory disease will be:

(1) cough,
(2) dyspnoea (breathlessness),
(3) sputum production (and/or haemoptysis),
(4) chest pain,
(5) cyanosis (blue discoloration of face, lips and fingertips),
(6) clubbing of the fingertips.

(A) RESPIRATION RATE AND CHARACTER

Control of respiratory movements is maintained by a centre in the medulla of the brain. It is sensitive to carbon dioxide in the blood, excess of which stimulates respiration and to the blood oxygen level, lack of which (anoxia) further stimulates the breathing rate. A rapid rate is thus brought about by the demands of exercise, an alteration in blood gas levels, an increase in the metabolic rate (as in any generalized infection and fever) and generalized disease or disorder of the respiratory system. Dyspnoea means difficult breathing, an unpleasant awareness of the act of breathing. It is usually due to oxygen-lack, thus in acute respiratory disease such as pneumonia there may be rapid shallow breathing.

In chronic bronchitis and emphysema the mechanics of respiration, the bellows function of the lungs, has suffered and the patient is dyspnoeic and distressed. His rib cage lifts instead of expanding properly, and his respiratory efforts involve the use of the neck muscles rather than the diaphragm.

In lung fibrosis the patient is breathless on slight exertion, but not necessarily dyspnoeic at rest.

Dyspnoea may be due to the pain of pleurisy, the patient being afraid to take a deep breath.

Wheezing due to bronchospasm accompanies the breathlessness of asthma, and the patient has special difficulty in expiration.

Stridor is noisy inspiration from inflammation or obstruction of the larynx, trachea or large bronchi.

Periodic breathing or Cheyne–Stokes breathing is where a period of apnoea (no breathing) occurs, then, as carbon dioxide builds up in the blood, stimulation of the respiratory centre occurs and deep sighing respirations develop, followed again by apnoea.

Air hunger is continuous deep breathing due to stimulation of the respiratory centre by acidosis.

(B) CHEST SOUNDS (AUSCULTATION)

Through a stethoscope the characteristic sounds of wheezing or stridor, as above, are magnified, but over local areas of the chest crepitations can be heard where the bronchial passages and the lung tissue is inflamed (as in bronchitis or pneumonia). A pleural rub may be detected in pleurisy, or areas of the chest where all respiratory sounds are diminished when there is lung or lobar collapse in pneumonia or pneumothorax. A knowledge of the normal anatomy of the thorax is necessary to compare breath sounds side by side.

(C) CHEST X-RAY

This is an essential addition to clinical examination of the chest. A portable film may be taken in the ward if the patient is too ill to move to the X-ray department.

A tomogram is a special view focused on the lesion.

A bronchogram is an X-ray following injection of radio-opaque iodized oil through the mouth or larynx to outline the bronchi.

(D) SPUTUM EXAMINATION

Purulent sputum denotes infection.

Bacteriology (staining and culture), reports should be considered in the light of the clinical findings, and response to treatment.

A knowledge of the infecting organism and its sensitivity allows adjustment of treatment if necessary.

Cytology for malignant cells is possible in suspicious cases and especially useful if the sputum is blood-stained.

(E) PEAK EXPIRATORY FLOW RATE

This is measured by rapid exhalation into a peak flow meter – it indicates the 'bellows' efficiency of the lungs and is impaired in airways obstruction, chronic bronchitis, and asthma.
The normal rate is 500 litres per minute.

(F) BLOOD GAS ANALYSIS

Arterial blood specimens are examined for their oxygen and carbon dioxide content, expressed as $P\text{O}_2$ and $P\text{CO}_2$ respectively. The effect of changes in these on the acidity of the blood is measured as the pH.

(Further special investigations would include laryngoscopy, bronchoscopy, spirometry and ventilation perfusion tests).

Common Disorders of the Respiratory System

(1) INFLUENZA

Cause

The influenza viruses. These have recently spread in epidemics from the Far East. Thus influenza virus A2, Hong Kong strain, caused epidemics in Britain in 1968 and 1970. The diagnosis is relatively easy during recognized epidemics. In non-epidemic years, the term 'influenza' is often vaguely applied to any febrile illness of uncertain cause.

Symptoms and signs

Fever.

Headache.

Cough.

Sore throat and catarrh.

Often of sudden onset and associated with limb pains and prostration.

Influenza-like illness, not necessarily due to the same virus, may be associated with conjunctivitis and running eyes, and sore throat.

Complications

Complications include bronchitis and pneumonia; these are a serious hazard in those with existing respiratory disease.

(2) DISORDERS OF THE LARYNX

Acute laryngitis may complicate a cold or respiratory infection, and present hoarseness, with cough and sputum.

Croup in children is due to laryngo-tracheo-bronchitis, caused by a virus, but superadded bacterial infection may seriously aggravate the disorder.

Angioneurotic oedema, an allergic reaction to something inhaled, ingested, or injected, may be so severe as to cause laryngeal oedema and obstruction.

Chronic laryngitis occurs in auctioneers and those who overuse the voice, especially if working in dusty atmospheres. It causes hoarseness and chronic cough.

Carcinoma of the larynx may also present with hoarseness so it is important to perform a laryngoscopy plus biopsy in suspected cases.

(3) ACUTE TRACHEITIS AND BRONCHITIS

Cause

Spread of the infection, usually bacterial from the upper respiratory tract after a cold or influenza.

The inflammation of the mucous membrane may involve the smallest bronchi, and spread into the alveoli and surrounding lung, when the condition becomes a bronchopneumonia.

Symptoms and signs

Fever.

Cough with moderate mucoid or purulent sputum.

Substernal discomfort.

(4) CHRONIC BRONCHITIS AND EMPHYSEMA (CHRONIC OBSTRUCTIVE AIRWAYS DISEASE)

In northern climates chronic bronchitis is a common and disabling disease; it is an inflammation of the small bronchi and bronchioles resulting in chronic cough and sputum.

The swelling of the bronchial mucous membrane causes narrowing and obstruction of the airflow, especially on expiration.

Emphysema is due to distension and destruction of the lung alveoli from the air-trapping in chronic bronchitis.

Causes

Cigarette smoking is by far the most important cause.

Atmospheric pollution with smoke and sulphur dioxide, especially in damp foggy climates, plays a part.

Bronchitis is more common in certain occupations, e.g. coal mining, from the effects of the inhaled dust.

Hereditary factors contribute, for a family history is common.

Infection causes flare-ups of the condition. While infection may initially be viral, bacterial infection follows, the organisms being commonly *Haemophilus influenzae* and the *Pneumococcus* (*Streptococcus*) *pneumoniae.*

Symptoms and signs

Chronic cough and sputum.
Breathlessness.

The mechanics of breathing are disturbed, the patient lifting his chest instead of expanding it on inspiration, and a 'barrel-shaped' chest may occur in emphysema.

Relapses are usually due to superadded infection, with increased cough, the sputum becoming purulent and increased in volume, and fever.

Severe relapses are characterized by cough, sputum, dyspnoea and cyanosis.

(5) BRONCHIECTASIS

Bronchiectasis is a dilatation with some destruction of the bronchial walls, associated with chronic infection. Localized dilatations occur which may be filled with pus.

Causes

May follow childhood whooping cough.

Conditions where mucus plugs or an inhaled foreign body cause bronchial obstruction. (The air is absorbed in the alveoli beyond the obstruction, causing areas of lung collapse. The surrounding healthy and elastic lung causes traction on the affected part, resulting in bronchial dilatation.)

Chronic bronchitis.

Pneumonia.

Symptoms and signs

Cough and the production of large quantities of purulent sputum.

'Dry' bronchiectasis may present as haemoptysis, sometimes massive.

Signs include 'moist sounds' heard with the stethoscope over the affected part of the lung.

Finger clubbing occurs.

(Diagnosis may be confirmed by bronchogram, the radio-opaque oil outlining the affected bronchi on X-ray.)

(6) PNEUMONIA

Pneumonia is an infection and inflammation of the alveoli of the lung. The infection is usually bacterial, but virus invasion of the respiratory tract may be a predisposing factor.

Pneumonia results in impaired oxygenation of the blood and various degrees of toxaemia.

Legionnaires' disease – a severe pneumonia recently found to be due to a small bacillus. (The first epidemic was reported from an American Legion convention in Philadelphia in 1976.)

The disease is spread through the inhalation of water droplets contaminated with the bacillus (as in showers).

Types

(a) *Lobar pneumonia* – a whole lobe becomes solid –consolidation usually caused by pneumococcus, sometimes by staphylococcus.

(b) *Broncopneumonia* – scattered areas of consolidation in one or both lungs. When there is infection and retained secretions in the smallest bronchi, the air in the related alveoli becomes absorbed causing patchy collapse and infection of the lung substances. Thus bronchopneumonia includes:

pneumonia following spread of respiratory tract infection;
aspiration pneumonia, where it is assumed infected matter has been inhaled;
hypostatic pneumonia – a complication of bed rest in elderly patients with cardiac failure or cerebrovascular disease, often a terminal event;
postoperative pneumonia – from failure to clear secretions (but some cases are pulmonary infarction).

(c) *Virus pneumonia* – pure virus pneumonia without secondary bacterial infection is rare, but may occur in influenza.

The organism *Mycoplasma pneumoniae*, not a true virus, may cause outbreaks of mild pneumonia in young adults. Organisms of the group *Chlamydia* (which have the characteristics of both viruses and bacteria) cause *psittacosis* in birds such as parrots and budgerigars, and *ornithosis* in pigeons. Human infection may occur in those in contact with such birds, causing a type of pneumonia.

Symptoms and signs

The onset is sudden with shivering and rigor followed by fever.

There is a harsh cough productive of a little 'rusty' sputum, later purulent.

Breathlessness.

Pleuritic pain.

Cyanosis.

Rapid pulse.

Toxaemia may be severe with delirium, hypotension and circulatory collapse.

(7) PULMONARY TUBERCULOSIS

Cause

Infection of the lung with *Mycobacterium (Bacillus) tuberculosis.*

Infection is acquired from inhalation of droplets or dust from the sputum of a person suffering from the disease. The source in developed communities of infection is usually a neglected elderly person, or a vagrant or alcoholic, or an immigrant from an underdeveloped country where tuberculosis may be rampant.

Primary infection may cause few symptoms (malaise, erythema nodosum) or pass unnoticed. Failure to heal may cause miliary spread. There may be healing with post-primary reactivation or reinfection involving a small part of the lung, or spreading to cause tuberculosis pneumonia, or the infection may become chronic; there is lung destruction with caseation (formation of cheesy material) and calcification, cavitation and fibrosis.

Persons with chronic tuberculosis form the important reservoir of infection and X-ray campaigns are directed towards detecting them.

(It is a wise precaution to have a chest X-ray of a patient with chest symptoms and living in poor circumstances, before admitting him to the general medical ward. A patient with a history of pulmonary tuberculosis who develops a chest infection should also be assumed to have a recrudescence of tuberculous infection until proved otherwise.)

Symptoms and signs

There may be none in the early stages, the diagnosis being made on chest X-ray.

Cough with sputum which may be mucoid or purulent.

Haemoptysis.

Fever and night sweats.

Weight loss.

(8) ASTHMA

Bronchial asthma is a condition characterized by recurrent attacks of wheeze and breathlessness. Attacks are due to airways obstruction from bronchial muscle spasm, and mucosal swelling and secretions.

Types

Asthma has recently been classified into two clinical groups: extrinsic asthma and intrinsic asthma.

Extrinsic asthma

Onset is in childhood and there is often a family history of a predisposition to allergic disorders including asthma, hay fever, eczema and skin sensitivity. The term extrinsic is used because an external allergen often precipitates an attack. The child or adolescent is symptom-free between attacks, which often become less frequent in adult life.

Precipitating factors include:

(a) *Allergy* – an allergic reaction to a substance following inhalation, ingestion or skin contact.

House-dust is a common allergen, probably due to the presence of a mite which feeds on the scales shed from human skin, and is found in mattresses and bedding. Feathers; the hairs from cats, dogs and horses; and moulds may also provoke asthma attacks.

Pollens are important allergens in the spring and early summer. Simple contact with plants such as certain primulas and foods such as shellfish affect some subjects.

(b) *Infection* – such as a cold or other respiratory infection.

(c) *Exposure* to cold air.

(d) *Psychological* factors – emotional upset such as anger, a broken love affair or domestic crisis (sometimes added to the above factors) precipitates many an attack of asthma.

Intrinsic asthma
This affects those over 40, wheeze persisting after a chest infection, and allergic factors may be less obvious. The patient may never be free of wheeze, and attacks tend to become more frequent and severe.

Symptoms and signs
Acute wheeze.

Distress with dyspnoea.

'Tightness' of the chest. (The chest tends to become fixed in inspiration, for the obstruction mainly affects expiration. The patient feels he cannot get his breath out, and he may be anxious with a fear of death.)

Cough, with the difficult expectoration of viscid sputum, but the sputum may be purulent if there is an infective basis for the attack.

Status asthmaticus with extreme dyspnoea, cyanosis, confusion and exhaustion – the picture of respiratory failure; in such cases the bronchioles may be plugged with viscid, rubbery secretions, and there is danger of death.

(9) CANCER OF THE LUNG (BRONCHOGENIC CARCINOMA)

Over two-thirds of patients die within a year of the diagnosis being made, and the overall 5-year survival rate is only 5%.

Causes
The malignant growth arises in a bronchus, and spreads to involve the lung lymph glands and distant organs, by metastatic spread by lymphatics or bloodstream.

Most cases are caused by heavy cigarette-smoking (25 or more a day).

Irritant and 'carcinogenic' substances in tobacco smoke may act by promoting malignant change in predisposed individuals. The incidence of lung cancer declines in those who stop smoking.

Atmospheric pollution plays a minor part.

Symptoms and signs

There are none in the early stages, the diagnosis being made on chest X-ray.

Middle-aged men are chiefly affected; there is dry cough and sometimes haemoptysis.

Sputum may become purulent from infection; bronchial obstruction causes breathlessness and partial collapse of the lung, pneumonia or lung abscess.

There may be finger clubbing.

Weakness and weight loss are late signs.

Complications

Pneumonia, lung abscess, pleural effusion.

Obstruction of the superior vena cava from spread to the mediastinum, causing pain, plethora and swelling of the face and neck.

The recurrent laryngeal nerve may be involved, causing hoarseness. Metastases in liver with jaundice, or in the brain with neurological or behavioural signs.

Metabolic effects, including neuropathy with sensory loss and weakness in the limbs, and ataxia (balance disturbance).

Endocrine effects include a low salt state and hypotension, and the opposite state from salt-retention, with Cushingoid features, the tumour producing an ACTH-like hormone.

(10) COLLAPSE OF THE LUNG (ATELECTASIS)

The term atelectasis is used to describe lung collapse following blockage of a bronchus. Lung collapse also occurs when air enters the pleural cavity (pneumothorax) and may rarely be caused by a massive pleural effusion.

Causes

A large bronchus may be blocked by an inhaled foreign body or retained secretion postoperatively. The air distal to the obstruction is absorbed, and the affected lobe or lung collapses.

The same process may occur less acutely when carcinoma obstructs a bronchus.

Patchy collapse affecting smaller segments of lung again occurs postoperatively, or in states of coma from retained mucus due to inadequate depth of respiration, and failure to cough effectively.

Symptoms and signs

If a lobe, or a whole lung is involved, there is sudden dyspnoea and cyanosis.

In small areas of collapse there may be only slight breathlessness and the symptoms and signs are those of pneumonia.

There is dullness to percussion and diminished breath sounds over the affected part.

X-ray changes including raising of the diaphragm from shrinkage of the lung. (Pulmonary embolism and infarction may cause a similar picture, sometimes with pleural pain and haemoptysis.)

(11) SPONTANEOUS PNEUMOTHORAX

Pneumothorax is the presence of air in the pleural cavity, causing partial or complete collapse of the underlying lung.

Causes

Rupture of a lung alveolus. While a distended area of lung in emphysema, an emphysematous 'bulla', may be responsible, in most cases the underlying lung is normal and the reason for the occurrence of pneumothorax obscure.

Symptoms and signs

The condition is commonest in young men, and may occur when quietly at rest or on respiratory effort in running or blowing a wind instrument.

DIFFERENTIAL DIAGNOSIS OF COUGH

	Severity	*Character*	*Productivity*
Chronic bronchitis	variable – mild in summer, severe in winter	paroxysmal at times; more marked during night or on rising	tenacious mucoid or mucopurulent sputum
Bronchogenic carcinoma	mild at first, may become severe	frequent but usually not paroxysmal	mucoid or mucopurulent sputum; non-productive at times
Pulmonary tuberculosis	becomes severe	initially dry and hacking; frequent but usually not paroxysmal	mucopurulent sputum (often green)
Bronchiectasis	Variable – mild, moderate or severe	prolonged paroxysms; more marked on rising, lying or bending	copious purulent sputum
Pneumococcal lobar pneumonia	mild at first; becomes severe	paroxysmal at times	sputum tenacious, mucoid and 'rusty'; become loose and mucopurulent
Acute tracheobronchitis	severe in pertussis and influenza	paroxysmal at times in influenza	maybe copious mucoid sputum, productive at times in influenza

Presence of blood	*Associated signs and symptoms*	*Main investigation findings*
haemoptysis uncommon	progressive exertional dyspnoea; roughened breath sounds; transient expiratory wheezes; fine moist râles; paranasal sinusitis and posterior rhinitis often present	X-ray normal or reveals increased hilar markings; emphysematous changes
blood-streaked sputum; frank haemoptysis common	weakness; malaise; chest pain; weight loss; anaemia; hoarseness; localized wheezing	X-ray – new density or mediastinal widening, without calcification (diagnosed by bronchoscopy)
haemoptysis common (massive haemorrhage occasional)	fever; night sweats; weakness; weight loss; fine and medium moist râles, mostly over upper lung; cavernous breath sounds over cavities	tuberculin test positive; sputum or gastric culture positive; X-ray will show patchy infiltrates with areas of fibrosis or cavitation
some haemoptysis common	fever absent; medium or coarse moist râles and rhonchi; amphoric breath sounds over dilated bronchi; clubbing of fingers may occur; intermittent pneumonia	sputum with pus cells; dilatations on bronchogram diagnostic
'rusty' sputum (degraded blood); frank haemoptysis uncommon	marked fever and prostration; headache; dyspnoea; cyanotic at times; pleuritic chest pain; signs of consolidation and moist rales over involved lobe; pleural friction rub	X-ray shows opacity of involved lobe; pneumococci often cultured from sputum and blood
haemoptysis rare	fever; generalized aching in influenza; coryza, rhinorrhoea and conjuncti-vitis in influenza and measles	very marked leukocytosis in pertussis; leukopenia often in influenza; positive culture in pertussis

DIFFERENTIAL DIAGNOSIS OF DIFFICULTY IN BREATHING: DYSPNOEA

	Dyspnoea	*Character of breathing*
Laryngitis/tracheitis	persistent; usually only on inspiration	prolonged, noisy inspiration
Emphysema	at first exertional; persistent in advanced cases	prolonged expiration; audible wheezing ronchi
Pneumonia	persistent	rapid and shallow; jerky expiratory grunting in lobar form
Bronchial asthma	paroxysmal with acute attacks	prolonged expiration; audible wheezing
Pneumothorax	persistent	rapid; shallow

Associated signs and symptoms	*X-ray changes*
usually barking painful cough; loud inspiratory stridor; hoarseness	X-ray normal
usually non-productive cough, may be productive on awakening; cyanosis may be marked; fixed chest	X-ray shows hyperlucent lung fields, depressed diaphragm
severe harsh cough, mucopurulent sputum; cyanosis may be marked; signs of consolidation, marked pleuritic pain and prostration in bacterial lobar pneumonia	X-ray shows diffuse bilateral density of lung tissue in pneumonias; opacification of consolidated lobe in bacterial lobar pneumonia
cough – at first non-productive, then sticky mucoid sputum; cyanosis may be marked; prolonged high-pitched expiratory sounds and wheezes; often sneezing	X-ray shows normal or hyper-inflated chest; eosinophils in sputum and blood
cyanosis; decreased breath sounds; tracheal deviation; hyperresonance on affected side	X-ray shows 'gas' in peripheral lung area

DIFFERENTIAL DIAGNOSIS OF CHEST PAIN ON BREATHING

	Character	*Location*	*Duration*
Acute pleurisy	sharp and jabbing only on breathing	lower lateral chest	usually few days
Pneumonia	sharp and jabbing only on breathing	over involved lobe; usually lower lateral chest	several days
Lung abscess	usually sharp and jabbing only on breathing; at times dull and aching	over abscess	several days
Pneumothorax	sharp and jabbing; may be continuous; intensified by breathing	lower axilla or under scapula	hours to days
Cancer	sharp and jabbing only on breathing; also dull and aching with tumour mass	over lesion or course of involved segmental nerve	few days; prolonged with tumour mass

Breathing	*Cough*	*Associated signs and symptoms*
shallow and rapid (proportional to pain)	non-productive	fever; pleural friction rub
severely dyspnoeic	severe and hacking; sputum blood stained or purulent	fever; pleural friction rub; râles; signs of consolidation; (pain prominent in bacterial pneumonia; not a feature of diffuse viral pneumonia)
shallow (proportional to pain)	copious sputum, purulent, often foetid and/or bloody	fever; pleural friction rub; râles; dullness to percussion; may follow aspiration
persistently dyspnoeic	ordinarily absent	diminished breath sounds; tympanitic or flat to percussion
shallow (proportional to pain); dyspnoeic with obstructive pneumonia	frequent with bronchial lesion	pain of rib fracture reproducible; râles with obstructive pneumonia and abscess

Sudden severe pain or discomfort as something is 'felt to give' and breathlessness. (Breathlessness usually improves in a few minutes, except on the rare occasions when the opening between lung and pleural cavity is valvular, allowing air in but not out, and causing 'tension' pneumothorax.)

Most cases are relatively mild and the patient may delay seeking medical advice. Examination reveals poor expansion on the affected side, and hyper-resonance on percussion.

(12) DISORDERS OF THE PLEURA

PLEURISY AND PLEURAL EFFUSION

Pleurisy is inflammation of the pleural membrane and may be 'dry' or accompanied by pleural effusion – fluid in the pleural cavity.

Causes

Usually there is underlying disease:

Lobar pneumonia.

Pulmonary infarction.

Lung cancer or pleural metastases.

Tuberculosis.

Rarer causes are virus infection of the chest wall and collagen diseases such as rheumatoid arthritis.

In effusion, the fluid may be an inflammatory exudate, containing cells and protein, or a transudate, a watery fluid formed as a reaction to the underlying disease.

Pleural effusion may accompany oedematous states such as heart failure, nephrotic syndrome and cirrhosis of the liver.

Empyema is a collection of pus in the pleural cavity; it may complicate lobar pneumonia from spread of pneumococcal infection, but is rare with effective antibacterial therapy.

Symptoms and signs

Pain, worse on deep breathing, occurs in dry pleurisy due to the rubbing-together of the inflamed surfaces and a 'pleural rub' may be heard with the stethoscope.

Large effusions cause breathlessness.

Dullness on percussion over the effusion.

In empyema, the patient is usually toxic and ill, with a swinging fever.

Further investigations

Chest X-ray confirms the presence of fluid.

Diagnostic aspiration of fluid – clear and straw-coloured if transudate.

May be cloudy if infected, or pus with empyema.

Blood-stained often in carcinoma and sometimes in pulmonary infarction.

Chapter 5
The Gastrointestinal System

Gastrointestinal diseases are the cause of more than 10% of all hospital admissions and medical consultations. Acute infections such as gastroenteritis are the commonest cause of medical consultation; appendicitis the commonest cause of emergency surgery; and carcinoma of the stomach, large intestine or rectum the most frequent cause of death from diseases of this system. In the young gastroenteritis can be lethal; in the mature patient gastrointestinal disturbance is a frequent cause of chronic disability, and in the elderly malignant disease of the system causes 10% of all deaths.

Diagnosis of disorder will depend on symptoms, history, observation of the patient and examination of:

(A) weight and fluid balance, diet and output chart;
(B) X-rays: e.g. using contrast medium (as in barium meal, swallow and enema);
(C) visualization of specifically affected part: e.g. oesophagoscopy, gastroscopy, sigmoidoscopy, proctoscopy;
(D) biopsy;

(E) bacteriology (stool samples, etc.);
(F) blood tests (for electrolyte levels and anaemia, etc.);
(G) examination of the mouth.

Common symptoms of gastrointestinal disease will be:

(1) anorexia,
(2) indigestion,
(3) nausea, vomiting and/or diarrhoea/constipation,
(4) pain,
(5) vomiting or passing of blood,
(6) loss of weight.

(A) WEIGHT

The body weight of the patient at the time of the illness, compared to either previous known weight or standard tables (see table) indicates the extent and duration, or effect, of the disease. Weight loss may be crucial in the newborn from the dehydration of gastroenteritis; in the chronically suffering patient weight loss may indicate a malignant disease and give objective assessment for the complaint of anorexia. Fluid balance, input and output charts are essential for assessing medication or i.v. needs in the vomiting patient.

(B) X-RAYS

Straight abdominal X-rays reveal gas levels in obstruction; contrast media X-rays reveal partial obstruction, dilatation, ulceration or disorders in the normal anatomy of the oesophageal, gastric, duodenal or intestinal outline.

(C) VISUALIZATION

Due to the benefits of fibre-optics, gastroscopy for example, along with other similar investigations, are much more easily and effectively performed than ever previously. They can all now be performed as outpatient procedures and enable the physician to undertake a biopsy of the apparently disordered tissues.

HEIGHT/WEIGHT TABLES FOR ADULT MEN AND WOMEN

Height (in shoes) *ft ins*	*Small frame* *lbs*	*Medium frame* *lbs*	*Large frame* *lbs*
	ADULT MEN		
5 2	112–120	118–129	126–141
5 3	115–123	121–133	129–144
5 4	118–126	124–136	132–148
5 5	121–129	127–139	135–152
5 6	124–133	130–143	138–156
5 7	128–137	134–147	142–161
5 8	132–141	138–152	147–166
5 9	136–145	142–156	151–170
5 10	140–150	146–160	155–174
5 11	144–154	150–165	159–179
6 0	148–158	154–170	164–184
6 1	152–162	158–175	168–189
6 2	156–167	162–180	173–194
6 3	160–171	167–185	178–199
6 4	164–175	172–190	182–204
	ADULT WOMEN		
4 10	92– 98	96–107	104–119
4 11	94–101	98–110	106–122
5 0	96–104	101–113	109–125
5 1	99–107	104–116	112–128
5 2	102–110	107–119	115–131
5 3	105–113	110–122	118–134
5 4	108–116	113–126	121–138
5 5	111–119	116–130	125–142
5 6	114–123	120–135	129–146
5 7	118–127	124–139	133–150
5 8	122–131	128–143	137–154
5 9	126–135	132–147	141–158
5 10	130–140	136–151	145–163
5 11	134–144	140–155	149–168
6 0	138–148	144–159	153–173

Weights include indoor clothing

(D) BIOPSY

Microscopic sections of tumour, gastric or intestinal wall, serve to diagnose the cause of the disorder.

(E) BACTERIOLOGY

Bacteriology of stool samples, as well as testing for the presence of blood and intestinal parasites, reveals the presence of infective organisms and indicates the necessary treatment.

(F) BLOOD TESTS

To assess the anaemic or infective status, and the physiological status (e.g. electrolytes, liver function tests, etc.), blood tests are an important part of the patient's profile.

(G) EXAMINATION OF THE MOUTH

The inspection of the tongue and the mouth is as important as the examination of the pulse.

The mouth reveals local pathology and the effects of many general conditions. Adequate fluids, the flow of saliva and the mechanical cleansing action of mastication, plus sound teeth and gums, contribute to a healthy mouth. It is an important part of the nurse's duty to encourage and maintain proper oral hygiene. Before the patient opens his mouth, conditions of the lips such as herpes simplex virus infection and accompanying febrile conditions may be noted. Cracks at the corners of the mouth (angular cheilitis) are as likely to be due to ill-fitting dentures as to poor nutrition or vitamin B deficiency.

The normal tongue is moist with somewhat rough surface from the papillae on it. A dry tongue implies mouth-breathing or dehydration. A light coating is normal, fur being normally removed by food and saliva. A furred tongue may simply indicate that the tongue is not being used much; marked furring occurs in heavy smokers, and in uraemia (renal failure). A smooth tongue (glossitis) is an atrophy of the papillae. A smooth pale tongue suggests anaemia, and in pernicious anaemia (vitamin B_{12} deficiency) the tongue may be sore. A fiery red or magenta tongue occurs in other B vitamin deficiencies, sometimes due to intestinal malabsorption. The tongue may show a tremor in alcoholism or Parkinson's disease. Carcinoma of the tongue may present as a painful, non-healing hard ulcer.

Dental decay (caries) is very common. Bacterial action on sugary foods and sweets produces acids which destroy the enamel, especially if sweets are eaten between meals and brushing of the teeth is neglected. Fluoride in the water supply is protective. In adults, periodontal disease with inflammation at the gum margins (gingivitis) is common, and there may be a mixed bacterial infection. Severe bleeding after dental extraction suggests a disorder of blood clotting such as haemophilia.

Bleeding of the gums occurs in scurvy (vitamin C deficiency) and in purpura and blood disorders such as leukaemia (excessive white cells) and agranulocytosis (lack of white cells), where there may also be ulceration.

Long-term treatment with phenytoin in epileptic patients may lead to swollen, hypertrophic gums. In lead poisoning, a blue line forms on the gums.

Stomatitis is inflammation of the mucous membrane of the mouth. There are many causes; prolonged fever and generalized illnesses with poor nutrition and lack of oral hygiene contribute to its development.

Thrush is an infection with the fungus *Candida (Monilia) albicans* and occurs where immunity is lowered, often in patients who have had steroids or broad-spectrum antibiotics such as tetracycline which destroy bacteria but allow monilia to flourish. There are white patches on a sore inflamed mucous membrane; removal of these fungal patches leaves a raw bleeding surface. The tongue, gums and throat may be involved.

Aphthous ulceration is recurrent crops of shallow ulcers of uncertain cause, often related to emotional stress.

Mouth ulceration occurs in skin diseases such as lichen planus and in blood diseases such as leukaemia and angranulocytosis.

Common Disorders of the Gastrointestinal System

(1) DYSPHAGIA (DIFFICULTY IN SWALLOWING)

The oesophagus (gullet) is a muscular tube about 25 cm (10 in) long connecting the pharynx with the stomach and lying for much of its course in the mediastinum behind the root of the lung and the heart. It ends just below the diaphragm at the 'cardia', the name given to the junction of oesophagus and stomach.

Causes

Painful conditions of the mouth and throat.

Swallowed foreign body.

Carconoma of the oesophagus, or involvement by extrinsic growths.

Stricture from corrosive fluids or following reflux oesophagitis and hiatus hernia.

Failure of relaxation of the muscle at the lower end of the oesophagus from atrophy of nerve endings here.

Neurogenic causes, such as bulbar palsy, or after strokes.

Emotional – the 'lump in the throat' feeling, at times of stress.

Myasthenia gravis, a rare condition with muscle weakness.

Symptoms and signs

In any form of obstruction, the patient can usually point accurately to its site.

The swallowing of solids becomes progressively more difficult; ultimately only liquids can be passed.

There is considerable loss of weight and emaciation.

Attempts at swallowing are followed by regurgitation of the food.

Following a stroke there may be transient dysphagia, but only after bilateral upper motor neurone involvement is there persistent disturbance of the swallowing mechanism, with risk of regurgitation of food into the lungs.

Further investigations

These include barium swallow X-ray, oesophagoscopy and biopsy.

(2) HIATUS HERNIA AND REFLUX OESOPHAGITIS

A hiatus is an opening, and a hernia is a protrusion of a viscus known in lay terms as a 'rupture'. In hiatus hernia, part of the stomach slides up through the diaphragmatic hiatus, or less commonly rolls up alongside the oesophagus, into the thorax. If the sphincter between stomach and oesophagus becomes incompetent, reflux of acid gastric juice has an irritant effect on the mucous membrane of the lower oesophagus causing oesophagitis, and stricture in severe cases.

Symptoms and signs

Heartburn and retrosternal pain.

Feeling of fulness and flatulence.

Symptoms are worse on lying down or stooping.

Acid regurgitation, vomiting and dysphagia may occur.

Anaemia may be due to oozing of blood from erosion or ulceration.
Barium X-ray shows the hernia, or allows demonstration of reflux.

(3) GASTRITIS

The stomach is a muscular organ which breaks up and mixes food; the mucous membrane contains cells secreting hydrochloric acid and pepsin which contribute to digestion.

Acute gastritis is an inflammation of the mucous membrane of the stomach.

Causes

Ingestion of irritant substances such as alcohol, aspirin.

Food poisoning. There is discomfort or pain, nausea and vomiting, usually settling in a day or two if further irritation is avoided.

(4) PEPTIC ULCER

(A) ULCERATION

A peptic ulcer is a hole in the mucous membrane of a part of the gastrointestinal tract to which gastric juice, hydrochloric acid–pepsin, has access.

Types

Gastric ulcer occurs in the stomach usually on the lesser (inner) curvature.

Duodenal ulcer occurs in the first part of the duodenum, just beyond the pyloric outlet of the stomach.

Causes

Peptic ulcer tends to run in families, suggesting a genetic predisposition.

The mucous membrane is normally resistant to the action of hydrochloric acid and pepsin. Ulceration occurs when the acid–pepsin versus mucosal resistance balance is disturbed. In duodenal ulcer there is a high acid–pepsin production from excess secreting cells in the stomach. In gastric ulcer the acid secretion may be high or low, and decreased mucosal resistance may be more important.

Mucosal resistance is lowered by heavy cigarette-smoking, alcohol, and certain drugs. (Thus aspirin may cause acute erosions and bleeding; phenylbutazone and indomethacin, used in the treatment of rheumatoid arthritis, cause gastric ulceration though persons with chronic diseases such as rheumatoid arthritis may have lowered mucosal resistance.

Factors such as overwork and mental stress cannot be proved to be causative, but they may exacerbate ulcer symptoms.

Symptoms and signs

The chief symptom is pain, felt in the epigastrium, and the patient may be able to point with one finger at its site, where there may be tenderness and resistance to palpation, with muscle 'guarding'.

It occurs between meals, is relieved by food and alkalis and often occurs in the middle of the night, around 2 a.m., waking the patient from sleep.

It has a characteristic periodicity, occurring over a few days or a week; then the patient may remain symptom-free for weeks or months.

Vomiting.

Haemorrhage and perforation.

Melaena.

Further investigations

Barium meal X-ray and screening shows an ulcer crater or duodenum deformity.

Gastroscopy (and duodenoscopy) using the flexible fibre-optic instrument permits a direct view with little discomfort to the patient, allows biopsy of gastric ulcer if malignancy is suspected and is indicated in all cases of X-ray negative dyspepsia.

(B) COMPLICATIONS

A haematemesis is a vomiting of blood which may be fresh and red or dark brown and 'coffee-ground' in appearance if altered by stomach acid.

A melaena is a loose, black, tarry, glistening stool from blood altered by passage through the alimentary tract, but if the haemorrhage is severe the stool may contain dark red blood.

Haematemesis and melaena

Causes

Gastric or duodenal ulcer eroding a blood vessel, and rarely gastric carcinoma.

Aspirin ingestion, often with another irritant such as alcohol. (Aspirin provokes bleeding from an existing peptic ulcer and in addition causes acute erosions, often multiple with oozing of blood.)

Cirrhosis of the liver with bleeding from oesophageal veins.

Bleeding states, caused by anticoagulants, or in purpura and leukaemia.

Haematemesis should be differentiated from haemoptysis (where the blood may be brighter and frothy), from a vomit of swallowed blood from a nose bleed, and from the vomiting of gastric contents in pyloric stenosis. If there is doubt, specimens must be preserved; their volume gives some indication of the severity of the haemorrhage.

Symptoms and signs

Bleeding may present as haematemesis, melaena or both, or may be 'silent' into the alimentary tract. The signs are those of blood loss:

Pallor.

Cold and clammy skin.

Apprehension and restlessness.

Rapid pulse and low blood pressure.

Fainting or collapse.

Dehydration from fluid loss.

Usually there is no pain, but there may have been an exacerbation of ulcer symptoms a few days previously.

Perforation

Cause

The ulcer erodes through the wall of stomach or duodenum with escape of gastric contents into the peritoneal cavity, causing severe irritation and peritonitis.

Symptoms and signs

Sudden severe upper abdominal pain.

Tenderness and board-like rigidity of the abdomen.

Rapidly rising pulse.

X-ray shows gas below the diaphragm.

Pyloric spasm and stenosis

Acute exacerbation of the ulcer may be associated with muscle spasm, so that the stomach does not empty properly and distends. In chronic ulceration there may be fibrous contraction at the duodenum beyond the pyloric outlet of the stomach, pyloric stenosis, with gross hold-up and distension.

Symptoms and signs

The ulcer pain changes its characteristics, now occurring after meals or in the evening when the stomach is distended.

Increasing weight loss, dehydration, salt and acid loss, and alkalosis on blood testing.

Gastric aspiration shows residual volumes of ½–1 litre; barium meal confirms gastric distension.

(5) CARCINOMA OF THE STOMACH

This occurs in the middle-aged and elderly. It should be suspected in non-healing gastric ulcers.

Symptoms and signs

Upper abdominal pain or discomfort not clearly related to meals.

Loss of appetite.

Weight loss.

Nausea and vomiting.

Mass may become palpable in the epigastrium.

Anaemia from blood loss.

The first signs may be of metastatic growths in the liver causing enlargement and jaundice, or in the peritoneal cavity causing ascites (fluid distension).

Further investigations

Early diagnosis is essential and is aided by:

Barium meal.

Gastric biopsy and gastroscopy.

Stool tests for occult blood, which may be positive.

Small intestine

The small intestine consists of the duodenum, and the jejunum and ileum lying in coils attached to the posterior abdominal wall by the mesentery (a fold of peritoneum in which blood vessels and lymphatics run). The ileum ends in the caecum; the start of the large intestine (colon) at the right iliac fossa.

The small intestine is concerned with digestion and absorption of foods, minerals and vitamins, the mucosa being in folds or villi which greatly increase the absorptive area. Enzymes secreted by the mucosa split food protein into amino acids; carbohydrates and sugars into glucose; these are absorbed into the blood vessels which join to form the portal vein to reach the liver. Fats are digested by the action of bile salts and pancreatic lipase, absorbed into lacteals in the villi to reach the lymphatics, and are carried via the thoracic duct to join the general circulation in the great veins near the heart.

The terminal part of the ileum contains patches of lymphoid tissue, Peyer's patches, which become involved in typhoid infection. The lymphoid tissue may be concerned in the body's immunity mechanism and the production of antibodies, and viruses may colonize here before spreading to other tissues, e.g. poliomyelitis.

(6) GASTROENTERITIS

This is caused by bacterial toxins, *Clostridia*, *Salmonella* and other infections. They include typhoid and paratyphoid (enteric fever), food poisoning, dysentery and cholera.

TYPHOID AND PARATYPHOID

Cause

Bacillus typhoid, and *B. paratyphoid* A, B and C (milder infection). These organisms belong to the *Salmonella* group.

Mode of infection

Faecal contamination from a patient or carrier, who may be symptomless. Water and foods such as meat products and milk transmit the infection where hygiene is poor.

Symptoms and signs

Typhoid is initially a bloodstream infection and during the first week the symptoms are not gastrointestinal, but systemic ones:

Fever.

Pulse slow in relation to the temperature.

Headache.

Weakness.

Fatigue.

Rose-spot rash of the abdomen.

There is constipation rather than diarrhoea at this stage and diagnosis may be difficult unless the condition is borne in mind.

Blood culture is positive during the first 10 days, and white cell count shows decreased polymorphs, instead of the increase in most infections.

If the condition is allowed to proceed, the patient becomes extremely ill with diarrhoea, pea-soup stools, abdominal distension and risk of bowel haemorrhage and perforation. Stool culture is then positive.

Diagnosis may be confirmed by the Widal agglutination test, which demonstrates the presence of the antibodies that develop after 2–3 weeks.

FOOD POISONING

Causes

Salmonella organisms:

Campylobacter organisms (from poultry and cattle) have recently been implicated in human enteritis.

Bacillus (Clostridium) welchii.

Staphylococcal – from preformed toxin.

Botulism.

The food poisoning *Salmonella* are pathogens of men and animals, and poultry, so that infection is acquired from human and animal cases, and meat and poultry products such as improperly cooked broiler chickens.

Symptoms and signs

These organisms are not invasive like the typhoid ones and cases present with gastric or intestinal symptoms rather than generalized disease, about 24 hours after infection:

Abdominal pain.

Vomiting and diarrhoea.

Fever and malaise.

Clostridium welchii grows in improperly cooked or reheated meat and symptoms start usually with diarrhoea 8–24 hours after ingestion.

The staphylococcal toxin is formed when the organisms multiply in food contaminated with pus from a food handler with a boil or abscess, or staphylococcal nasal discharge, and vomiting occurs 2–5 hours after the infected meal.

(7) DYSENTERY

BACILLARY DYSENTERY

Cause

Bacilli of the *Shigella* group, of which *Sh. sonnei* is much the commonest, though other organisms cause more severe dysentery, especially in the tropics. They are purely human pathogens, causing inflammation of the large bowel (colon).

Mode of infection

From the faeces of cases, and carriers, usually by the hands, from objects such as lavatory seats. This is how *Sonnei* dysentery spreads in nursery schools, where infection is common, and in hospital wards. Contamination of food and water may cause epidemics.

Symptoms and signs

Lower abdominal discomfort.

Fever and diarrhoea often with blood mucus in the stools.

Malaise from toxaemia in severe cases.

AMOEBIC DYSENTERY

This is due to bowel infection with the small parasite *Entamoeba histolytica*, which occurs in the tropics and spreads in cystic form from the stools. There is diarrhoea with bleeding and bowel ulceration, but the symptoms may be mild. There may be spread to the liver, causing amoebic abscess, which may discharge through the diaphragm and be coughed up as pus. A fluorescent antibody test in the blood may be helpful.

CHOLERA

This disease is caused by a bacillus (*Vibrio*) spreading by contamination of water supplies. It is a fulminating bowel infection, with copious fluid 'rice-eater' stools.

CROHN'S DISEASE (REGIONAL ILEITIS)

This is a relapsing inflammatory disorder of areas of the small intestine, usually the terminal ileum; the colon and anus may also be involved. The cause is unknown but there is a familial incidence, the disease affecting mainly young adults.

Symptoms and signs

Abdominal pain.

Diarrhoea.

Lack of appetite.

Weight loss and fever.

Acute episodes may simulate acute appendicitis with pain and tenderness at the right iliac fossa.

May be intestinal obstruction with vomiting and a palpable mass or peritonitis.

The stools may contain blood or be fatty (steatorrhoea) with malabsorption from the lower ileum.

Anaemia.

Diagnosis may be confirmed by narrowing of terminal ileum on barium 'follow-through'.

(8) MALABSORPTION SYNDROME

This is a group of conditions in which absorption of foods through the small intestine is impaired. Fat absorption is especially impaired, but carbohydrates, proteins, minerals and vitamins are also poorly absorbed, in varying degree.

Steatorrhoea means frequent, pale, greasy, bulky and offensive stools which float in the toilet and are difficult to flush away.

Causes

Lesions of the small intestine

Coeliac disease occurs in children (failure to thrive, 'pot-belly' and rickets).

Coeliac syndrome or idiopathic steatorrhoea is the adult equivalent. These conditions are due to an intolerance to the protein fraction called gluten in wheat and rye flour.

Tropical sprue occurs in certain zones especially in the Far East, but may persist on return to temperate climate.

Crohn's disease and infiltrations of the intestine in conditions such as Hodgkin's disease and blood disorders, tuberculosis, and amyloidosis also cause malabsorption.

Lack of digestive enzymes or bile salts

E.g. chronic pancreatitis and obstructive jaundice. Intestinal lactase deficiency is of importance in causing failure of digestion of lactose (milk-sugar) with resultant intolerance to milk.

After surgical operations

E.g. gastrectomy, massive resections of intestine, and with

'blind-loops' which often harbour bacteria which utilize nutrients and impair digestive action.

The parasite *Giardia lamblia* may cause malabsorption in children.

Symptoms and signs

Steatorrhoea.

Weight loss.

Anorexia and distended abdomen.

Anaemia is a common presentation from deficiency of iron, folic acid and vitamin B.

Other vitamin B deficiencies cause sore red tongue and peripheral neuritis.

Osteomalacia (the adult equivalent of rickets) due to lack of vitamin D and calcium, causes bone thinning and fractures.

Bleeding tendency due to lack of vitamin K.

Oedema and ascites due to hypoproteinaemia.

Low blood potassium causes further general weakness.

Further investigations

Faecal fat estimation – stools are collected for 3–5 days on a normal ward diet; with steatorrhoea, faecal fat output exceeds 6 g per 24 h.

Glucose tolerance test – in malabsorption the blood sugar curve is 'flat' after 75 g oral glucose, but the test is not reliable in chronic pancreatitis where there may be associated diabetes.

Xylose absorption test – xylose is a sugar which in normal people is absorbed but not metabolized so it is excreted unchanged in the urine. In malabsorption, 25 g is given by mouth and less than 20% appears in the urine in 5 h.

Barium meal and follow-through shows a 'clumping' pattern.

Intestinal biopsy – a small metal capsule attached to a thin plastic tube, is swallowed, preferably in the evening so as to pass into the small intestine by the next morning, its position being verified on X-ray. A syringe is attached to the tubing (which has been fixed at the mouth) and suction triggers off a tiny cutting edge in the capsule, into which a minute piece of intestinal mucosa is drawn. The device is then slowly withdrawn through the mouth, and the biopsy specimen examined. In coeliac disease and some of the other conditions, the villi are deformed and flattened.

Other investigations are directed towards the anaemia and include serum levels of iron, folic acid and B_{12}.

Mineral lack may be detected by serum calcium, phosphorus and alkaline phosphatase tests, and by X-rays of bones. The serum potassium may be low. Protein deficiency results in a low serum albumin.

The large intestine (caecum, colon and rectum)

The large intestine starts at the caecum (from which protrudes the appendix) in the right iliac fossa, then becomes the ascending, transverse and descending colon, and pelvic or sigmoid colon, rectum and anal sphincter. The external muscular layer is collected into three longitudinal bands which are shorter than the rest of the colon, causing puckering or 'haustration'. The function of the colon is the absorption of water and minerals, converting the intestinal contents to semisolid faeces (about 150 g daily). The rectum is normally empty, faeces entering causing stimulation and defaecation of the pelvic and descending colon contents. The colon normally contains *Escherichia coli* and large numbers of other bacteria which may cause serious disease in tissues outside the colon.

(9) CONSTIPATION

Constipation is the infrequent and difficult passage of hard faeces. Most people have a bowel action daily, normal 'habit-time' being after breakfast as the result of the gastrocolic reflex stimulus. There is, however, considerable variation, some people normally having a motion only three or four times per week.

Causes

Failure to answer the call to stool – this may be due to inadequate time at breakfast, lack of toilet facilities, forced use of the unpleasant bedpan, or physical weakness in the elderly. Fluid becomes absorbed from the stools in the rectum, resulting in hard motions or faecal impaction.

Abuse of purgatives – after powerful purgation, the whole colon may empty, take a day or two to refill so that further purgation is taken to attempt to produce a motion. The bowel may become dependent on such stimulation, and true constipation follow its withdrawal.

Dietary – a large part of the faeces is in fact of non-dietary origin; however, inadequate bulk in the diet and lack of fluids may cause constipation.

General illness, especially febrile illness, and bed rest with lack of exercise is a possible factor. Depressive states and myxoedema (hypothyroidism) are also causes.

Disorders of the colon

Carcinoma: change in bowel habit, i.e. constipation in someone previously regular, should raise suspicions.

Adhesions after operation.

Anal fissure making defaecation painful.

Symptoms and effects

The only symptoms of constipation are vague loss of appetite and abdominal discomfort, due to distension.

Constipation is, however, important in the elderly for it may result in faecal impaction in the rectum and spurious diarrhoea, a little watery faeces being squeezed past the obstruction; impaction may also cause both faecal and urinary incontinence.

A heavy loaded colon may press on pelvic veins, worsening varicose veins in the leg, and possibly contributing to venous thrombosis. Urinary tract infections may be commoner if there is constipation, the mode of infection being uncertain.

Straining at stool worsens haemorrhoids and is undesirable in those with cardiac and respiratory disease.

(10) DIARRHOEA

Diarrhoea means the passage of frequent or loose stools. After defaecation in some cases there may be a residual feeling of unsatisfactory evacuation or 'tenesmus'.

Causes

(A) Acute

(1) Gastrointestinal infections
- (a) food poisoning, as part of gastroenteritis;
- (b) typhoid and paratyphoid;
- (c) dysentery – stools contain blood and mucus, and are often watery;
- (d) cholera – profuse 'rice-water' stools with little faecal matter.

(2) Melaena from bleeding peptic ulcer, aspirin ingestion, or oesophageal varices – stools loose, black and tarry.

(3) Excessive use of broad-spectrum antibiotics such as tetracycline, which cause upset in the normal bowel bacterial flora.

(B) Recurrent or chronic

(1) Small intestine
- (a) malabsorption syndrome – steatorrhoea (fatty stools);
- (b) Crohn's disease – stools loose and may contain blood, or steatorrhoea.

(2) Large intestine
- (a) irritable colon syndrome;
- (b) diverticular disease;
- (c) ulcerative colitis;
- (d) carcinoma.

(3) General causes
anxiety and 'nerves';
thyrotoxicosis (hyperthyroidism);
diabetes – nocturnal diarrhoea;
pellagra (a vitamin B factor, nicotinamide, deficiency).

Further investigations

The stool must always be inspected, and sent for bacteriological investigation if there is any suspicion of an infective cause. Occult blood tests and faecal fat estimation may also be required; sigmoidoscopy, barium enema or barium meal and follow-through.

Effects of diarrhoea

Severe diarrhoea is debilitating (and may be fatal in infants). Large amounts of fluid, sodium and potassium may be lost leading to hypovolaemia, hypokalaemia, and collapse. Nutrients are lost in the steatorrhoea of malabsorption, and blood in melaena.

(11) IRRITABLE COLON SYNDROME (SPASTIC COLON)

This is an ill-defined disorder presenting as frequency of bowel movement, or urgency after meals – suggested causes include over-active gastrocolic reflex, intestinal hurry from lactase deficiency (when removing milk from the diet may help) and disturbance of motility of the large bowel, and anxiety.

(12) DIVERTICULAR DISEASE OF THE COLON

Diverticulosis is the presence of little 'pouchings' of mucous membrane through the muscular wall, where blood vessels enter, of the pelvic and descending colon.

Causes

A disturbance of motility, often with muscle thickening.

Chronic low-grade infection, related possibly to chronic anxiety and tension.

Related to lack of bulk (fibre) in the diet, for the disorder is rare in underdeveloped countries.

Symptoms and signs

Abdominal discomfort.

Colicky pain at the left lower abdomen.

Altered bowel habit.

Episodes of constipation or large bowel obstruction.

Distension and later vomiting.

Tenderness, fever and malaise.

A mass may become palpable from peri-diverticular abscess, and there may be perforation with peritonitis, or fistula formation.

Further investigations

These may include barium enema; sigmoidoscopy.

(13) ULCERATIVE COLITIS

This is an inflammatory disease of the large intestine. It may be confined to the rectum and pelvic colon, or the whole colon may be involved. There is patchy ulceration and bleeding of the mucous membrane, and in late stages fibrosis and shortening of the bowel. Ulcerative colitis occurs in young and middle-aged adults and is slightly commoner in women.

Cause

The cause is unknown.

'Autoimmunity' has been suggested; the body destroying its own tissues. Some patients have been found to have antibodies to cows' milk in their blood and a few patients have lactase deficiency in the small intestine, but in most cases milk sensitivity seems to have little bearing on the condition.

Psychosomatic factors have been involved – these include tense personality, insistence on precision and tidiness, and repression of emotional feelings, the bowel 'losing its temper' instead.

Symptoms and signs

Episodes of diarrhoea, often with blood and mucus in the stools, which may amount to about a dozen loose motions daily.

Tenesmus (persistent desire to defaecate) and the patient is afraid to go far from a toilet.

(There are remissions in which bowel movement may return towards normal but relapses tend to occur over months or years.)

Fulminating attacks of bloody diarrhoea are associated with fever, emaciation and anaemia.

Complications

Complications include bowel abscess, stricture and perforation. Where the whole colon is involved, toxic dilatation and rupture may occur, and in long-standing cases there is an increased risk of carcinoma. Ulcerative colitis may also have systemic complications including skin sepsis and abscesses, erythema nodosum, arthritis (which may involve spinal joints), spondylitis, iritis, liver inflammation and cirrhosis, and a tendency to venous thrombosis.

Further investigations

Stool bacteriology – to exclude infections.

Sigmoidoscopy – this is an examination through the rectum. The mucosa is red, granular and bleeds easily and there may be mucus or a mucopurulent exudate.

Barium enema shows an irregular or ulcerated mucosal pattern, loss of haustrations, and in late stages a tube-like colon. Straight X-ray may show toxic dilatation in acute cases.

Blood examination may show anaemia, raised white cell count and ESR, and fluid and electrolyte depletion, especially a low potassium, from prolonged diarrhoea.

(14) CARCINOMA OF THE RECTUM AND COLON

Carcinoma of the large bowel is common (causing some 15 000 deaths annually in Britain) and therefore being second only to carcinoma of the bronchus in terms of mortality from cancer. The disease is most frequent in the middle-aged and elderly, but can occur in young people.

Symptoms and signs

Cancer of the rectum is commonest, symptoms include:

Bleeding (often mistakenly ascribed to piles);

Change of bowel habit, often with diarrhoea and passage of slime;

The cancer may be palpable with the finger on rectal examination (cancer of the pelvic colon presents similarly);

In the descending and transverse colon, the change of bowel habit is likely to present as constipation rather than diarrhoea, and there may be stricture and obstruction with abdominal distension and later vomiting;

Growths in the caecum and ascending colon may be silent, the complaint being of vague deterioration in health, weight loss, and weakness from anaemia due to occult bleeding;

A mass may become palpable in colonic cancer in later stages;

Sometimes the growth presents as metastases in the liver with jaundice, or as ascites.

Further investigations include stool tests for occult blood, sigmoidoscopy and barium enema. Blood examination may show anaemia and raised ESR. Laparotomy (surgical exploration of the abdomen) may be indicated in suspicious cases even when barium enema is negative.

(15) THE ACUTE ABDOMEN

When confronted with a patient with abdominal pain and vomiting, the decision as to whether the condition is a 'surgical' one requiring operation may not be possible without careful observation and charting of pulse and temperature. Diabetic ketosis may present with abdominal pain and vomiting, operation is lethal in this situation, and the urine must be routinely tested for sugar and ketones to exclude it. Analgesics to relieve pain may obscure diagnosis of the acute abdomen, and should only be given when the course of management has been decided. In doubtful cases, it may be necessary to proceed to laparotomy.

(a) *Acute appendicitis* is commonest in children and young adults, but may occur in the elderly.

Symptoms:

central abdominal discomfort;

followed by pain, tenderness and muscle guarding at the right iliac fossa, slight vomiting;

raised pulse and temperature, but pyrexia may not be marked. (Mensenteric adenitis is an inflammation of abdominal lymph glands in children and may have similar symptoms.)

(b) *Perforated peptic ulcer* causes severe upper abdominal pain, tenderness and rigidity.

(c) *Acute cholecystitis, biliary colic* and *acute pancreatitis* cause abdominal pain.

(d) *Renal colic* causes pain in the loin or iliac fossa – these conditions are described in later chapters.

(e) *Ruptured ectopic pregnancy* is a 'gynaecological' emergency; pregnancy has occurred in the ovarian tube instead of the uterus, the tube ruptures in the early weeks causing severe lower abdominal pain and usually vaginal bleeding. There is a history of a missed period.

(f) *Salpingitis*, inflammation of the ovarian tubes, is another cause of lower abdominal pain.

(g) *Intussusception* is an invagination of one length of intestine into another; it occurs in infants, and in adults in association with a lesion such as a polyp or carcinoma.

Symptoms:

pain;

vomiting;

bloody diarrhoea;

palpable mass;

(h) *Intestinal obstruction* has many possible causes:

herniae caught at the inguinal and femoral canals;

adhesions from previous operations;

carcinoma;

mesenteric arterial thrombosis causing ischaemia and stasis;

volvulus (sudden twisting) of the bowel in the elderly.

Symptoms include pain and vomiting, but if the large

DIFFERENTIAL DIAGNOSIS OF VOMITING –

	Onset and duration	*Severity and frequency*
Obstructed ulcer	long after meals, often during night	initially frequent, not copious
Carcinoma of the stomach	gradual in onset; initially only after a heavy meal; often repeated bouts with free periods	may become intractable and severe
Alcoholic gastritis	begins during alcoholic excess of next morning; may last several days or only few hours	may be persistent and severe
Intestinal obstruction	sudden in onset; persistent until obstruction relieved	severe and frequent, especially with high obstruction
Biliary colic	sudden in onset	often recurrent and severe
Pancreatitis	sudden in onset, usually only an early symptom	usually not severe or persistent, but may persist if ileus develops
Appendicitis	an early symptom	usually not severe or persistent
Peritonitis	occurs early, and then recurs when ileus develops	initially forceful and severe; later meagre and frequent
Staphylococcal food poisoning	sudden, 5–6 h after food; lasts 4–6 h	severe and frequent; retching and salivation present

Due to Gastrointestinal Disorders

Associated findings	*Key laboratory findings*
reduction in typical ulcer pain; feeling of fullness, relieved by vomiting; thirst, oliguria, succussion splash of stomach	gastric aspirate – large volume and retained food particles; obstruction seen on barium studies of stomach; hypokalaemic alkalosis
epigastric pain; belching; feeling of fullness, weight loss, pallor, melaena often; palpable epigastric mass in some; metastatic nodes	may be visualized by X-rays and/or gastroscopy; cytological study of gastric washings may show tumour cells
headache, tremor, epigastric tenderness, haematemesis and melaena may occur	typical lesions seen on gastroscopy and gastroscopic biopsy
colicky epigastric or periumbilical pain, constipation, no flatus; may be weak and shock-like; abdomen soft until distended then diffusely tender; loud bowel sounds, visible peristalsis in some	X-ray shows fluid level in 3–4 h
pain in right upper quadrant and epigastrium, may radiate to right shoulder, causes patient to flex trunk; belching, cold sweats; fever and chills if cholangitis; jaundice at times; abdomen soft	radio-opaque stones on flat film in some; diagnosis often confirmed by cholangiogram
history of alcoholic excess, biliary disease or recent surgery; severe epigastric pain; wide-ranging temperature; tender epigastrium, slightly rigid or soft; shock in severe cases	leukocytosis, elevated serum amylase, often low serum calcium; X-ray may show calcified pancreas or distortion of duodenum
preceded by indigestion or flatulence; periumbilical colic at first in many; then continuous pain and tenderness in right lower quadrant; rebound tenderness and local rigidity in same area; sometimes local distension; rectal tenderness in many	leukocytosis; X-ray may show local distension
finding of precipitating illness; high fever usual; severe pain initially diffuse, then often more localized; intense and rebound tenderness, diminished or absent bowel sounds; distension may develop	leukocytosis; X-ray shows ileus and intraperitoneal fluid
colicky periumbilical or hypogastric pain; diarrhoea, at times bloody; sweating, prostration, rarely shock; little or no abdominal distension or tenderness	temperature normal, no leukocytosis; diagnosis by smear or culture

DIFFERENTIAL DIAGNOSIS OF DIARRHOEA – 1

	Onset and duration	*Severity*	*Character*	*Nature of stool*
Salmonellosis	sudden; usually 2–5 days; occasionally up to 4 days	mild or severe	straining and tenesmus may be present	stools watery with increased mucus;
Shigellosis	sudden; may last 2–10 days	severe – 20 or more movements a day	straining and tenesmus	watery, greenish, with increased mucus; blood and pus in severe cases
Amoebiasis	usually gradual; sudden at times; chronic or recurrent	mild or severe; frequent, small bowel movements	tenesmus in many	small, liquid or semiliquid, with bloody mucus
Cholera	abrupt	usually severe	no tenesmus or abdominal cramping	stools watery, profuse, flecks of mucus – no blood or pus – 'rice water'
Staphylococcal enterocolitis	sudden; often persists unless treated; death may occur in 24–48 h	mild, or severe and continuous	often 'explosive'	may be soft with faecal material, or watery green with blood
Viral enteritis	sudden or gradual – lasts from 1 day to a week	mild or severe	tenesmus uncommon	watery diarrhoea; no blood, mucus or pus
Ulcerative colitis	usually gradual; can be abrupt in fulminating form; few weeks to chronic	from 2–3 to 15–20 movements a day	often nocturnal; often tenesmus, urgency, rectal incontinence	soft and mushy or loose, bloody, mucoid – pus in most severe
Regional enteritis	gradual, continuous or recurrent	from 2 to 10 stools a day	nocturnal at times; tenesmus uncommon	stools soft, semiliquid; watery in very severe; bloody pus with colonic disease; bulky foul stools with small bowel disease

Abdominal findings	*Associated signs and symptoms*	*Key laboratory findings*
increased peristalsis; tenderness	abdominal cramping, nausea and vomiting present; fever; chills; toxic	diagnosis by culture of stool; leukopenia in some
increased peristalsis; abdominal tenderness, especially over colon	cramping may be first symptom; nausea, vomiting, fever – variable	sigmoidoscopy – red, oedematous mucosa with pinpoint and larger ulcerations; diagnosis by culture of stool
may simulate acute appendicitis	may be very toxic with fever and chills; anaemia, malnutrition, lethargy	leukocytosis marked in acute; no eosinophilia; sigmoidoscopy – small, punched-out ulcers; exudate may show parasites or cysts
abdomen often soft; no tenderness	vomiting late, without nausea; muscular cramping; thirst, cyanosis, shock; hypotension; poor skin turgor	marked haemoconcentration, often renal shutdown and uraemia; organisms in stool identified by agglutination or culture
distended, with diminished bowel sounds in severe cases; mild, diffuse tenderness	often begins after antibiotics; high fever in some; toxic, drowsy, confused; nausea, vomiting, hiccups; abdominal pain mild or absent; signs of shock in some	haemoconcentration, hypokalaemia, hyponatraemia, hypochloraemia, acidosis; stool smear and culture on blood agar will show staphylococci; sigmoidoscopy will show sloughing
audible borborygmi; mild abdominal tenderness; increased peristalsis	cramping is prominent; fatigue and dry mouth at onset; malaise, anorexia, nausea; vomiting usually only at onset; fever in some; headache, dizziness; flatus increased; weakness, dehydration	bacterial flora of bowel normal on culture; blood count and chemistry usually normal
tenderness over left colon; peristalsis usually normal; some distension	cramping abdominal pains – left lower quadrant; backache; rectal bleeding; weakness, anorexia; nausea; nervous; fever in some; anal sphincter spastic, often haemorrhoids and fissures	sigmoidoscopy – varying degrees of bleeding erythema, ulceration; findings at barium enema diagnostic; often hypoalbuminaemia and anaemia – no leukocytosis
tender mass in right lower quadrant common; may simulate appendicitis; signs of bowel obstruction at times	periumbilical cramps, often relieved by defaecation; bloating, flatulence; back pain; fever at times; rectal and anal fistulae; melaena uncommon	sigmoidoscopy – ulcerations in some; barium enema shows colonic involvement, often segmental; stricture formation at times; anaemia and hypoproteinaemia

DIFFERENTIAL DIAGNOSIS OF DIARRHOEA – 2

	Onset and severity	*Character of diarrhoea and stools*	*Gastrointestinal symptoms*
Gluten enteropathy	gradual; chronic; variable in severity	less than 10 movements a day; usually bulky, frothy, steatorrhoea, but may be watery	anorexia; distension, cramps, flatulence
Sprue	gradual or acute; chronic or recurrent	often 'explosive', may awaken patient; stool soft, bulky, pale – steatorrhoea	anorexia; nausea and vomiting at times; flatulence, borborygmi
Chronic pancreatitis	gradual chronic; moderate in severity	usually steatorrhoea; may be watery	previous episodes of acute abdominal pain, often of biliary disease
Cystic fibrosis	gradual; chronic; moderate	3–6 movements per day; steatorrhoea, almost never watery	appetite increased, except during infections; variable abdominal pain
Carcinoma of rectum	gradual; chronic or recurrent; usually not severe	stool often small and deformed with mucorrhoea, mixed with blood; often urgency and sense of incomplete evacuation	pain during or after defaecation; constipation at times; rectal bleeding at times, independent of defaecation

Abdominal signs	*Associated findings*	*Key laboratory data*
some abdominal distension at times	weakness, weight loss, glossitis, skin and mucosal bleeding; dependent oedema in some; urine volume greater at night; tetany and paraesthesias at times	serum proteins low; anaemia; hypocalcaemia; cholesterol low; faecal fat increased; X-ray – dilated small bowel; segmentation and fragmentation of barium, thickening of folds; jejunal biopsy – shortening and thickening of villi
abdomen, often protuberant; anal sphincter lax	weakness, weight loss; pallor of skin and mucosa, glossitis, aphthous stomatitis	macrocytic anaemia; serum proteins low, often hypokalaemia; faecal fat increased; X-ray of small bowel shows 'sprue' pattern; small bowel biopsy – short, thick villi
tenderness or fulness of epigastrium in some; ascites in some	history of chronic alcoholism common; glossitis, weight loss	amylase and lipase elevated after acute attack; glucose tolerance test shows diabetic curve; faecal fat increased; X-ray may show calcification of pancreas
Abdominal distension in infants; prolapse of rectum	weight loss or retarded growth; obstructive respiratory symptoms; cough, copious sputum; prostration from salt depletion in hot weather, sweating increased	sweat shows increased sodium and chloride; faecal fat increased; chest X-ray-hyperinflation, often collapse of segment; small bowel X-ray – nutritional deficiency pattern
liver may be enlarged; tumour often palpable on rectal digital	weight loss and cachexia at times; dull perineal ache in some; urinary frequency or tenesmus in some	tumour visible via proctoscope; anaemia from blood loss; leukocytosis at times; elevation of SGOT and alkaline phosphatase with hepatic metastases

bowel is involved vomiting may not be marked and there is constipation. The abdomen becomes distended and 'fluid levels' are seen on X-ray.

(i) *Paralytic ileus* is an atony of the small intestine post-operatively or complicating intestinal obstruction or peritonitis. Secretions continue to be poured into the intestine, which is unable to pass its contents onwards or to absorb them. The patient becomes increasingly dehydrated, with hypotension and collapse. Nasogastric suction and intravenous fluids and antibiotics are required until the causative condition is relieved or intestinal motility is re-established.

(j) *Peritonitis* may complicate any of these conditions. The peritoneal membrane of the abdomen is similar to the pleural membrane of the thorax. The visceral layer of peritoneum covers the intestines and is not sensitive to pain, the parietal layer lines the abdominal wall and is pain-sensitive. The peritoneal cavity is the potential space between the two layers. A large fold of peritoneum called the greater omentum is spread like an apron over the intestines, separating them from the anterior wall of the abdomen.

Peritonitis is inflammation of the peritoneum and results from spread of inflammation from abdominal or pelvic organs.

Symptoms and signs:

- pain;
- tenderness and muscle guarding, which may remain localized by the 'policeman' action of the greater omentum, with subsequent healing or abscess formation;
- the peritonitis may become generalized with rapid pulse, pyrexia and toxaemia from infection.

(k) *Ascites.* Ascites is the presence of fluid in the peritoneal cavity.

Causes:

- *congestive cardiac failure* – part of the generalized oedema from fluid retention;
- *nephrotic syndrome* (renal disease with albuminuria and oedema);
- *cirrhosis of the liver* – ascites due to low plasma albumin and raised portal venous pressure, causing fluid exudation into the peritoneal cavity.
- *malignant ascites* – from peritoneal metastases in carcinoma of the stomach, large intestine or ovary.

Symptoms and signs:

- abdominal distension, but this is not marked in early stages;
- dullness to percussion over the flanks, the dullness shifting when the patient is asked to role to one side;
- increasing ascites will show the umbilicus becoming everted and the abdomen tense and uncomfortable:

Diagnostic tap may be required in suspected malignant ascites, a specimen of fluid being sent for cytology for malignant cells. The fluid may be blood-stained and often accumulates rapidly in such cases.

Chapter 6

The Digestive System (Liver, Biliary Tract and Pancreas)

Disorders of the organs involved in the digestive system are in general those that affect the adult, with the exception of infective hepatitis in the young. Gallstones are commoner in fertile females over 40 years of age than in men, cirrhosis of the liver is of increasing frequency in the adult male of mature years due to alcohol consumption. Pancreatic disease affects both sexes equally.

Diagnosis of disorder will depend on symptoms, history, observation of the patient and examination of:

(A) urine,
(B) blood tests,
(C) X-rays (including contrast media use and angiography),
(D) ultrasound scanning,
(E) biopsy.

Common symptoms of digestive organ disease will be:

(1) anorexia and nausea,
(2) jaundice,
(3) pain,
(4) fever,
(5) ascites (free fluid in the abdominal cavity).

(A) URINE TESTS

Bilirubin (pile pigment) gives a brown colour to the urine, and on shaking in a test-tube, the froth is yellowish.

Reagent strips confirm presence of bilirubin.

Urobilinogen is colourless and reagent strips may be used.

Acetone may be detected by odour and confirmed by reagent tablet or strip.

Sugar is detected by reagent strip test.

(B) BLOOD TESTS (e.g. liver function tests)

Test on venous blood include serum bilirubin, enzymes such as SGPT (raised in liver cell dysfunction) and alkaline phosphatase (raised in obstructive jaundice), proteins and prothrombin.

(C) X-RAY EXAMINATION

Cholecystography – the patient is given an evening dose of iodine-containing substance excreted by the liver into the bile: it becomes concentrated in a normal gallbladder, which will show up on X-ray next morning. Further films after a fatty meal will show contraction of a normal gallbladder and outline the bile duct. Straight abdominal X-ray may in certain cases show gallstones.

Percutaneous cholangiography – where X-ray contrast medium injected into the liver allows demonstration of a blocked biliary tree – may be of great help in localizing the site of an obstruction.

Portal venography is also useful diagnostically in certain particular diseases.

(D) ULTRASOUND SCANNING

This investigation shows abnormalities of the liver and biliary tract including blockage from stones and the presence of tumours. It is a non-invasive investigation, causing no discomfort to the patient. It is becoming established as a most useful early investigation in liver, gallbladder and pancreatic disease.

(E) LIVER BIOPSY

Using local anaesthetic, a special needle is inserted between the right lower ribs in the mid-axillary line, and passed into the liver from which a small specimen is withdrawn for microscopical examination. This investigation is contraindicated if the patient has a bleeding tendency or is severely jaundiced.

The liver, the largest organ in the body, is wedge-shaped, and occupies the uppermost right part of the abdomen immediately below the diaphragm, sheltered by the ribs. The portal vein carries to it the food products absorbed in the intestine, and it receives arterial blood from the hepatic artery.

The hepatic duct carries bile from the liver and joins the cystic duct from the gallbladder to form the common bile duct. This usually unites with the main pancreatic duct just before opening into the second part of the duodenum. The gallbladder is a pear-shaped bag on the under-surface of the liver, opposite the anterior end of the ninth costal cartilage. It stores and concentrates the bile.

Most of the liver cells are specialized hepatic cells, but the liver also contains cells of the reticuloendothelial system. The reticuloendothelial system includes cells in the spleen, liver, lymph nodes and bone marrow. It has a scavenger function for worn-out cells and foreign material, and a function in the immunity mechanism, producing the immune globulins or antibodies. Thus the liver may become involved in blood diseases such as leukaemia and Hodgkin's disease.

FUNCTIONS OF THE LIVER

(1) METABOLISM AND STORAGE

Carbohydrates are metabolized and glucose stored as glycogen. Proteins are synthesized from amino acids. Thus the liver makes plasma-albumin and prothrombin, which is necessary for blood coagulation; Vitamin K is required for its synthesis. In protein breakdown, ammonia is formed and is converted by the liver to urea which is excreted by the kidneys in the urine.

Fats are catabolized to fatty acids which provide a reserve

source of energy when glucose metabolism is upset as in diabetic ketosis. Vitamin D is partially hydroxylated and stored in the liver, with vitamins A and B.

(2) DETOXIFICATION

The liver renders harmless the body's waste products. It also destroys toxic substances and drugs, or conjugates them chemically to prevent their further action and allowing their excretion in the urine or, in some cases, into the bile.

(3) BILE SECRETION

The liver produces the bile salts, which by their 'detergent' action, cause the emulsification of dietary fats into small globules for digestion by pancreatic lipase in the intestine. Bile salts are necessary for the absorption of the fat-soluble vitamins A, D and K. Bile also contains bile pigment, bilirubin, which has no digestive function but gives bile its colour.

Bilirubin metabolism: the red blood cells become worn out in 120 days, when they are taken up by cells of the reticulo-endothelial system. The haemoglobin is broken down, iron is detached from the haem and retained for further use; the remainder of the haem molecule goes to form bilirubin. It is carried by the bloodstream to the liver where it is taken up by the hepatic cells.

Common Disorders of the Gastrointestinal Organs

(1) JAUNDICE

Jaundice is a yellow discoloration of the tissues due to excess bilirubin in the blood. Jaundice is often first noticed in the skin of the abdomen, or in the sclera (white part) of the eyes, but an observant nurse may note it in the plasma when reading an ESR.

TYPES

(a) Pre-hepatic – excessive production of bilirubin

This is haemolytic jaundice or haemolytic anaemia, from abnormal red-cell destruction (see Chapter 13, 'The blood and lymphatic system').

There is no bile in the urine. This is because bilirubin is not water-soluble when just formed from red cells. Because of the large amount of bilirubin reaching the colon in haemolytic jaundice, much urobilinogen is formed and reabsorbed, overwhelming the excretory capacity of the liver, so that an excess of urobilinogen appears in the urine.

(b) Hepatic

This is due to disordered function of the liver cells. It is caused by infections, such as hepatitis, poisons such as carbon tetrachloride (used in dry-cleaning and as a fire extinguisher) and benzene (a solvent), drugs and by some rare familial diseases. Depending on the degree of swelling and obstruction to bile outflow, the stools may be normal in colour or pale. Reabsorption of bilirubin rendered water-soluble by passage through the liver causes bile to appear in the urine. In the early stages of liver cell dysfunction, the capacity of the liver to re-excrete urobilinogen is one of the first functions to be impaired. Urobilinogen is at this stage detectable in the urine.

(c) Post-hepatic or obstructive jaundice

This is due to blockage of the bile duct by a stone from the gall-bladder, or by carcinoma of the head of the pancreas. The jaundice is deep and the skin often itchy. The stools are pale and clay-coloured, the urine dark brown from the presence of bile pigment, bilirubin.

Effect

The bilirubin in the tissues is not in itself harmful in adults. In haemolytic disease of the newborn (which is due to Rhesus factor antibodies) the excess bilirubin is toxic to the infant brain.

In obstructive jaundice fat digestion is impaired and vitamin K cannot be absorbed. Prothrombin manufacture may also be impaired by hepatic jaundice. Failure of blood coagulation and bruising tendency results.

Drugs and the liver

If liver function is impaired drugs normally destroyed by the liver may reach toxic concentrations in the bloodstream. Morphine and barbiturates (excluding phenobarbitone which is excreted unchanged in the urine) are such drugs and they must not be given to patients suffering from disorders of the liver.

(d) Jaundice due to drugs

The mechanisms of drug-induced jaundice are complex. Substances such as carbon tetrachloride, chloroform, and benzene are directly toxic, causing liver cell necrosis, and a very high concentration of tetracycline and paracetamol may have a similar effect. The anaesthetic halothane if used repeatedly, and the monoamine oxidase inhibitors, used in treatment of depressive illness, may cause a hepatitis-like jaundice. Chlorpromazine and its derivatives, oral contraceptives and sex hormones may cause a less severe sensitivity (cholestatic) jaundice, which clears when the drug is stopped.

(2) VIRUS HEPATITIS – INFECTIOUS HEPATITIS AND SERUM HEPATITIS

Cause

A virus present in the patient's stools and transmitted by faecal contamination of food or water is the cause. Cases may occur sporadically or in epidemics where hygiene is poor, and have followed the eating of shellfish from sewage-polluted waters.

The incubation period is about 30 days. Jaundice is the hallmark of the infection but may be mild, and many cases go undiagnosed. The faeces are infective from about 2 weeks before, to 2 weeks after, the onset of jaundice. Infectious hepatitis is commonest in children and young adults.

Serum hepatitis is also a virus infection from blood or blood products, infection is spread usually by blood transfusion or by injection from contaminated syringes and needles. The incubation period is up to 120 days. Adults are mainly affected, the illness frequently being more severe than infectious hepatitis.

The blood of some patients with serum hepatitis contains an antigen related to the presence of a virus called the hepatitis-B associated antigen, HbAg (or Australia antigen as it was first found in the serum of an aborigine). It may persist for many years due to a deficiency of the immunity mechanism and the blood is infective, although the carrier may be symptomless. This led to outbreaks of hepatitis in renal dialysis units. Though screening for this antigen diminishes the risk, other viruses may be responsible for cases of hepatitis: non-A, non-B hepatitis.

Drug addicts are at risk from contaminated syringes, and as hepatitis is common among homosexuals, secretions other than blood transmit the infection. (e.g. saliva).

The virus is destroyed by autoclaving or dry heat sterilization but a better preventive measure is the use of disposable equipment where possible, and the avoidance of blood transfusion unless there is a clear indication for its use.

Gammaglobulin prophylaxis

Injections of this immune globulin may prevent the development of infectious hepatitis after exposure in epidemics. This measure is indicated in pregnant women. Gammaglobulin prophylaxis is of less value in serum hepatitis.

Symptoms and signs

Loss of appetite.

Malaise and generalized aches.

Fever.

Nausea and vomiting occur.

Jaundice becomes manifest.

Abdominal discomfort with liver swelling and tenderness.

Fulminating cases develop deep jaundice and high fever and may go into hepatic failure and coma.

The stools become pale during hepatitis.

The urine may contain excess urobilinogen in the earliest stages, but with liver cell swelling and obstruction to bile outflow this disappears and the urine becomes dark due to the presence of bilirubin, which clears as the jaundice lessens.

Liver function tests in the blood are also abnormal.

Mental depression is often marked.

(3) CIRRHOSIS OF THE LIVER

Cirrhosis is diffuse fibrosis of the liver with areas of nodular regeneration. (The word cirrhosis is derived from a Greek word meaning tawny, the colour that the liver may acquire in this condition.)

TYPES

There are two main types: portal cirrhosis and biliary cirrhosis.

Portal cirrhosis is the commoner type and is a disease of middle-age. The patient is not usually jaundiced (except terminally), the trouble affecting the portal venous system, though the liver cells are also involved.

Biliary cirrhosis is associated with obstruction to bile outflow, which may be primary from intrahepatic disease or secondary from extrahepatic biliary obstruction, and the patients are jaundiced.

Primary biliary cirrhosis occurs in middle-aged women. The cause is unknown; like chronic active hepatitis, it may be a disturbance of immunity to hepatitis-associated antigen and certain antibodies are detectable in the blood. There is jaundice with dark urine and pale stools, and severe pruritus.

Secondary biliary cirrhosis occurs if bile duct obstruction from stone, stricture, or carcinoma goes unrelieved for months or years.

Portal cirrhosis

Causes

Alcoholism – the commonest cause in many countries.

Dietary deficiencies and effects of toxins and parasites especially in the tropics.

Following virus hepatitis.

Right sided heart failure and constrictive pericarditis if untreated.

Rare diseases with liver fibrosis – haemochromatosis from iron deposition in pancreas and liver, and hepatolenticular degeneration (Wilson's disease) from copper deposits in the liver and basal ganglia of the brain.

Symptoms and signs

Vague ill-health, anorexia and mild fever.

The finding of an enlarged liver and enlarged spleen. In portal hypertension, distension occurs where veins of the portal system anastomose with the systemic veins, causing varicose veins at the lower end of the oesophagus, dilated vessels in the abdominal wall near the umbilicus and splenic enlargement.

Haematemesis occurs from ruptured oesophageal varices, though bleeding may occur from peptic ulcer or gastric erosions commonly associated with alcoholism.

Anaemia is common.

Splenic enlargement may inhibit the release of cells from the bone marrow (which remains active) resulting in deficiency of platelets causing bleeding, and of white cells with increased susceptibility to infections.

In liver cell dysfunction the appearance of vascular spiders on the face, neck and arms may be seen. These are little red spots consisting of a dilated arteriole from which tiny vessels radiate.

The skin of the palms of the hands is pink, contrasting with the muddy colour of the skin as a whole in cirrhosis.

Ascites is common, from the combined effects of portal hypertension and reduced serum albumin in the blood. (Albumin normally maintains the osmotic pressure, the 'holding force' by which fluid is retained in the circulation. The leakage of fluid from the bloodstream to form ascites lowers the blood volume, and compensatory mechanisms to retain fluid in the body come into operation; these include secretion of the adrenal cortical hormone aldosterone which causes salt and water retention which further increases the ascites and causes oedema.)

Aldosterone also causes potassium loss with muscle weakness as a result.

Jaundice is a late sign, heralding liver cell failure, build-up of toxic nitrogenous substances causes depression of brain function or portal–systemic encephalopathy and coma.

Further investigations

The urine contains excess urobilinogen.

Liver function tests in the blood are abnormal, and the electrolytes, especially potassium, must be checked.

Liver biopsy may elucidate the type of cirrhosis.

Barium swallow demonstrates oesophageal varices.

Portal venography may be helpful.

(4) LIVER CELL FAILURE AND HEPATIC COMA

Hepatic failure with jaundice, bleeding tendency and the ill effects of increased circulating nitrogenous substances absorbed from protein breakdown in the intestine, leads to coma.

Causes

Acute liver poisoning and necrosis from chemicals such as carbon tetrachloride, benzene and chloroform; and halothane, paraquat, paracetamol poisoning and other toxins.

Fulminating virus hepatitis.

Cirrhosis of the liver. Precipitating factors include alcohol intake, intercurrent infections, gastrointestinal haemorrhage causing excessive protein load, and potassium deficiency.

Symptoms and signs

These are those of the causative condition, of which the commonest is:

Cirrhosis.

Increasing jaundice.

Fever and effects of the nitrogenous toxins.

There is a flapping tremor of the outstretched hands, lethargy and variable mental confusion.

The electroencephalogram (EEG) shows typical changes in the brain waves.

(5) SECONDARY CARCINOMA

The liver is a very common site of metastatic growths, spread by the portal or systemic veins from primary carcinomas in the abdomen, such as stomach and large intestine, or in the chest, such as carcinoma of the lung or breast.

Symptoms and signs

There may be evidence of the primary growth, but the secondary carcinoma in the liver may present first.

There is malaise, lassitude.

Weight loss.

Abdominal swelling: The liver may be huge and nodular.

Ascites from peritoneal metastases.

Jaundice may be mild or severe when major bile ducts are invaded.

The urine may contain bilirubin and/or urobilinogen.

(6) GALLSTONES AND THE BILIARY TRACT

Gallstones are formed when some of the constituents of the bile are deposited from solution. There may be excessive production of cholesterol by the liver. As bile is concentrated in the gallbladder, stones are most frequently formed here.

Gallstones occur at all ages, but are very common in middle-aged women who are obese and have borne many children – women who are fair, fat, fertile and forty. Hormonal effects on bile composition or gallbladder motility, and infection may be causative factors.

Symptoms and signs

May be symptomless, especially in the elderly.

Associated with cholecystitis.

Bile duct obstruction with colic, jaundice and cholangitis from infection of the stagnant bile.

(7) CHOLECYSTITIS

(a) ACUTE

This is acute inflammation of the gallbladder, usually associated with a gallstone obstructing the neck of the gallbladder or the cystic duct, and there is super-added infection often with *Escherichia coli.*

Symptoms and signs

Precipitated by a fatty or heavy meal.

Epigastric discomfort followed by severe pain and tenderness at the right upper quadrant over the gallbladder as the peritoneum becomes involved.

Pain may be referred to the right scapula or tip of the shoulder.

Anorexia, malaise and fever.

Occasionally vomiting but jaundice suggests bile duct obstruction.

The white cell count is raised.

Straight X-ray may show opaque stones.

(b) CHRONIC

This presents as recurrent attacks of acute cholecystitis, or as dyspepsia and upper abdominal discomfort often provoked by fatty foods or a heavy meal.

Thus the diagnosis of chronic cholecystitis must be confirmed by cholecystography, which shows gallstones and a poorly functioning gallbladder.

(8) BILE DUCT OBSTRUCTION

This is caused by a gallstone passing into the common bile duct, resulting in biliary colic, jaundice and cholangitis.

Symptoms and signs

Biliary colic is severe intermittent colicky pain or a more prolonged pain building up over an hour or two, felt in the epigastrium or right upper quadrant of the abdomen, and accompanied by vomiting.

Jaundice may be mild or deep and is obstructive in type with pale stools and dark urine, but the obstruction is rarely complete so that the stool colour may vary from day to day.

Cholangitis is inflammation of the bile duct from infection of the stagnant bile.

This causes fever, often of an intermittent type, accompanied by pain and jaundice.

Further investigations

These include blood culture, ultrasonic scan and cholangiography.

THE PANCREAS

The pancreas is an elongated gland that lies across the upper part of the posterior wall of the abdomen, its head in the loop of the duodenum, its body and tail extending to the left behind the stomach.

The gland cells secrete the pancreatic juice containing enzymes which act on protein, fat and carbohydrate. These enzymes are activated on meeting the duodenal juices. The main duct of the pancreas unites with the bile duct to form what is called the ampulla just before entering the second part of the duodenum. The sphincter surrounds the ampulla and prevents reflux of duodenal contents into the pancreatic duct.

The islet cells, or islets of Langerhans, secrete the hormone insulin into the bloodstream. Insulin is especially concerned with glucose metabolism, and deficiency of its action results in diabetes mellitus.

(9) PANCREATITIS

(a) ACUTE

Associated with disease of the biliary tract or gallstones – with alcoholism – reflux of duodenal contents into the pancreatic duct activates the enzymes resulting in self-digestion of the pancreas and necrosis of surrounding fat – an acute inflammatory process.

Symptoms and signs

Sudden agonizing upper abdominal pain.

Nausea and vomiting.

The abdomen is tender and rigid.

Pallor, rapid pulse and often hypotension and collapse.

Shock due to lowered blood volume from outpouring of fluid into the intestine.

The diagnosis of acute pancreatis is confirmed by a very high serum amylase, one of the enzymes that leaks into the bloodstream.

(b) CHRONIC

In chronic pancreatitis there is a gradual destruction of the pancreatic cells with replacement fibrosis and permanent impairment of function.

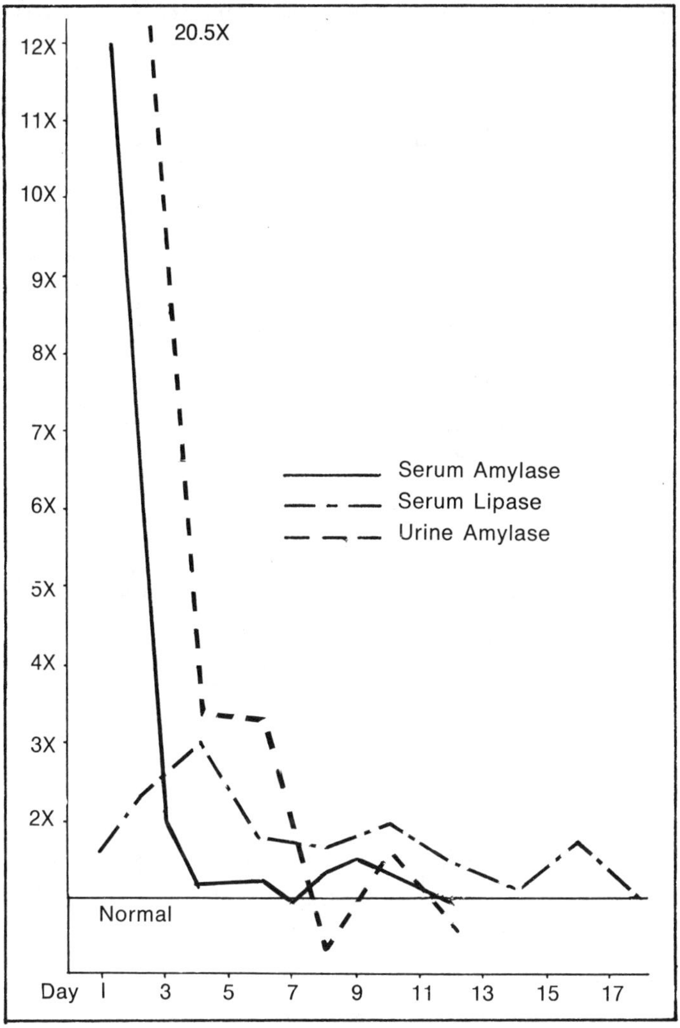

Amylase and lipase elevations in acute pancreatitis

Cause

The cause is often unknown, but alcoholism and dietary deficiencies may be responsible.

Sequel to acute pancreatitis or biliary tract disease.

A gallstone pressing on the pancreatic duct.

Carcinoma of the pancreas may also be associated.

DIFFERENTIAL DIAGNOSIS OF ABDOMINAL PAIN –

	Character	*Location*	*Produced or relieved by*
Peptic ulcer	gnawing, aching	in upper epigastrium, may radiate to back	precipitated by spicy or greasy food, anxiety; usually relieved by antacids or food; at times by vomiting
Perforated peptic ulcer	initially severe, continuous; then less severe but still continuous	at first epigastric, then generalized; may radiate to top of one or both shoulders	initial pain spontaneous, later pain made much worse by movement
Intestinal obstruction, small bowel	intermittent, colicky, persistent with distension or strangulation	epigastric and periumbilical; localized over strangulation when present	onset spontaneous and unpredictable
Intussusception	sudden onset, severe, intermittent – lasts a few minutes, recurs after minutes or hours	maximal in periumbilical region	vomiting may give give temporary relief
Intestinal obstruction, large bowel	onset sudden; colicky, each spasm less than a minute, comes at intervals of a few minutes	usually hypogastric, in midline	onset spontaneous

Due to Gastrointestinal Disorders

Abdominal physical findings	*Associated signs and symptoms*	*Key laboratory findings*
abdomen soft, but may show diffuse epigastric tenderness	nausea and vomiting common, appetite good – weight stable; retrosternal burning and increased salivation may occur; sour taste in mouth frequent; abdominal cramping on left side common – from associated irritable colon	may have iron deficiency anaemia, blood in stool; X-ray after barium will show ulcer crater
abdomen initially diffusely rigid, then tender; with peritonitis, rigidity goes, but still tender, becomes distended	preceding ulcer symptoms usually present; pale, sweating, weak pulse, shallow respiration – initially retching; hiccups	chest X-ray may show free air under diaphragm; leukocytosis present
abdomen soft until distension develops then generalized tenderness visible peristalsis of stomach or small bowel – loud bowel sounds, borborygmi – rebound tenderness	weak, shock, no fever until strangulation; vomiting – most prominent with high obstruction; constipation, dehydration and oliguria	X-ray of abdomen – fluid levels in 3–4 h
a sausage-shaped mass may be palpated in the abdomen – becomes firmer with pain; the right iliac fossa feels empty; signs of obstruction	usually one normal stool after onset, then bloody mucus and constipation; vomiting late	barium enema: one portion of bowel invaginated into another
distension early and marked; increased peristaltic sounds, more marked during pain	vomiting may not be present, but nausea is; constipation, no flatus	X-ray of abdomen – fluid levels in 3–4 h

(continued overleaf)

DIFFERENTIAL DIAGNOSIS OF ABDOMINAL PAIN –

	Character	*Location*	*Produced or relieved by*
Appendicitis	initial colicky pain in many, then persistent and continuous, of varying intensity	colicky pain in central abdominal area, continuous in right iliac fossa	made worse by extension of right thigh
Pancreatitis	severe, continuous, may last days to week	epigastric; radiates widely, often to back and/ or one or both loins; or to left scapular region	may accompany mumps or follow laparotomy; recurrent type often follows alcoholic excess
Cholecystitis	continuous – varies from mild to severe – present before nausea and vomiting	right upper quadrant and epigastrium; may be referred to right hypochond-rium and tip of right shoulder	worsened by breathing
Biliary colic	severe pain – crescendo for 20 min then gradually recedes	maximal in right upper quandrant or epigastrium, may radiate to right shoulder	slightly relieved by flexed posture
Diverticulitis	acute, continuous, may last several days; collicky pain, as well, at times, from partial obstruction	initially hypogastric, then then maximal in left iliac fossa; may radiate to low back	may be precipitated by large meals with much roughage or by strenuous exercise

Due to Gastrointestinal Disorders (cont'd)

Abdominal physical findings	*Associated signs and symptoms*	*Key laboratory findings*
tenderness – often rebound rigidity; superficial hyperaesthesia; audible borborygmi	often anorexia, indigestion and flatulence; diarrhoea precedes attack at times; some nausea and vomiting, but not persistent; fever and rapid heart rate; urinary frequency, tenesmus and rectal tenderness	leukocytosis always present
abdomen usually tender in lower epigastrium; either somewhat rigid or soft; marked rigidity is rare	retching – at times incessant – often bilious vomiting; fever; icterus at times; in severe cases – shock with cold, clammy skin – often purpuric staining of left flank and/or periumbilical region after several days	marked leukocytosis; serum amylase over 500 initially, may fall during attack; serum Ca^{++} may be reduced; X-ray – pancreas calcified in recurrent type
always local tenderness in right upper quadrant; often local rigidity	often history of biliary disease and fatty food intolerance; vomiting slight unless stones or peritonitis; usually constipated; some fever, more with cholangitis; usually no jaundice	leukocytosis always present; plain film of abdomen may show stone – cholecystogram will usually show nonfunctioning gallbladder
abdomen is soft – there may be deep local tenderness in right upper quadrant	often history of biliary disease or colic; much nausea and vomiting – bilious with retching, belching, cold sweat – patient appears near collapse; diarrhoea at times, fever and chills with cholangitis; jaundice in some	radio-opaque stones may be seen on flat film of abdomen; if no filling of gallbladder on intravenous cholangiogram, suspect blocked cystic duct (or severe liver disease); cholangiogram may show dilated common duct and location of stone(s)
guarding and local rigidity in left lower quadrant – vague mass may be palpable	long history of constipation, with diarrhoea at times; flatulence; prior rectal bleeding or bloody stools in most; nausea and vomiting; fever and tachycardia – may have rectal tenderness	leukocytosis usual; barium enema X-ray shows diverticula – irregular narrowing, wedge-shaped defects suggest diverticulitis

(continued overleaf)

DIFFERENTIAL DIAGNOSIS OF ABDOMINAL PAIN –

	Character	*Location*	*Produced or relieved by*
Ulcerative colitis	usually intermittent, colicky; continuous with acute dilatation or perforation	maximal in hypogastrium or left lower quadrant	often precipitated by emotional stress; often relieved by defaecation

DIFFERENTIAL DIAGNOSIS OF ASCITES –

	Time and speed of onset	*Amount of fluid*
Portal cirrhosis	gradual onset, but may be sudden; early in course	often massive
Post-necrotic cirrhosis	gradual onset; any time in course	variable, usually less than portal cirrhosis
Acute alcoholic hepatitis	gradual or sudden onset; usually early in course	variable, may be massive
Portal vein thrombosis	sudden onset; usually early in course	large to massive
Metastatic malignant liver disease	gradual onset; usually early in course	variable; rarely massive

Due to Gastrointestinal Disorders (cont'd)

Abdominal physical findings	*Associated signs and symptoms*	*Key laboratory findings*
abdomen usually soft, not tender – distended, tender with acute dilatation	diarrhoea frequently nocturnal, often bloody with muco-pus; tenesmus, fever, malaise; rectal – tight sphincter	WBC count normal, many toxic forms; alkalosis with low Na^+, K^+, Cl^- and protein; proctosigmoidoscopy – hyperaemia, granularity, purulent exudate, ulceration; barium enema – ragged outline, ulceration, narrowing, shortening, loss of haustration

Due to Hepatic Diseases

Other associated signs and symptoms	*Key laboratory findings*
weakness, fatigue, jaundice; right upper quadrant abdominal pain; gynaecomastia	liver function tests show non-specific abnormalities; occasionally hyperlipaemia with or without anaemia; diagnostic test – liver biopsy
weakness, fatigue, jaundice; often gynaecomastia and loss of libido; upper gastrointestinal bleeding may occur; palmar erythema, oedema	liver function tests often non-specifically abnormal; occasional abnormal serologic tests, LE phenomenon, hypergammaglobulinaemia; liver biopsy diagnostic
jaundice, fever, abdominal pain, dehydration; occasionally haematemesis; palmar erythema	liver function tests non-specifically and moderately abnormal; uric acid up, potassium down; occasional hyperlipaemia, anaemia which may be haemolytic
right upper quadrant abdominal pain; often nausea, vomiting, haematemesis, melaena in over 50%; oesophageal varices in more than 90%	liver function tests variable; occasional pancytopenia or isolated cytopenia; diagnostic test – splenoportography
cachexia – weakness, anorexia, fever; right upper quadrant abdominal pain; jaundice in some; occasional upper gastrointestinal bleeding	liver function tests – elevated alkaline phosphatase, SGOT; bilirubin sometimes high; often anaemia and leukocytosis; liver scan shows space-occupying lesion; liver biopsy usually diagnostic

Symptoms and signs

Bouts of upper abdominal pain, persistent and demoralizing, often precipitated by a heavy meal or alcohol.

Pain may be worse lying flat.

Slight jaundice, and fever.

Sometimes there is no pain, the condition presenting as pancreatic insufficiency with malabsorption syndrome from lack of digestive enzymes.

There is weight loss and steatorrhoea – loose, pale, offensive, fatty stools.

Diabetes in the late stages, from destruction of the insulin-secreting islet cells. There is polyuria and thirst.

Further investigations

Straight X-ray may show pancreatic calcification.

The serum amylase may be slightly raised.

Stools show a high fat content (normally less than 6 g/24 h).

Glucose tolerance test may show a high diabetic curve instead of the flat curve of intestinal causes of malabsorption, and xylose absorption is normal.

Ultrasonic and radioisotope scans prove helpful.

(10) CARCINOMA OF THE PANCREAS

This occurs in the middle-aged and elderly.

Symptoms and signs

The onset is insidious.

Upper abdominal pain similar to that in chronic pancreatitis.

Anorexia and weight loss.

Obstructive jaundice may be the first sign.

The jaundice is deep with itchy skin, pale stools and dark urine.

Metastases are frequently the first clinical indication – ascites from peritoneal deposits, or liver swelling.

Involvement of the inferior vena cava causes venous obstruction and oedema.

Further investigations

Barium meal may show distortion of the loop of the duodenum. The ESR may be raised, as in any malignant disease.

Ultrasonic and radioisotope scanning of the pancreas may be helpful.

Chapter 7
The Urinary System

The commonest disorder of the urinary system is acute infection. In primary care infection will be the most frequent cause of consultation for disorders of this system, but only 5% of hospital admissions will be due to disorders of the urinary system. Renal calculi, renal colic, nephritis, and renal failure will be the most frequent causes of hospital admission for diseases of this system, but they account for less than 1% of all deaths.

Diagnosis of disorder will depend on symptoms, history, observation of the patient and examination of:
(A) urine,
(B) blood and urine tests to determine renal function,
(C) X-rays (plain and contrast),
(D) cystoscopy,
(E) Renal biopsy.

Common symptoms of generalized disorder will be:
(1) dysuria and/or frequency,
(2) haematuria,
(3) pain,

(4) oedema,
(5) hypertension.

(A) EXAMINATION OF THE URINE

Appearance

Colour

The normal yellow or amber colour is due to urochrome. Dark urine may simply be concentrated urine or due to the presence of bile (bilirubin). Blood in the urine, haematuria, is either frank and obvious or causes a dark, 'smokey' urine.

Deposits

Urates form a brown or pink deposit when urine cools on standing. Phosphates are white and appear in neutral or alkaline urine. A cloud of mucus may be seen. These are normal findings and should be distinguished from pus in the urine, pyuria (which may be creamy and offensive) and from haematuria, but microscopic examination may be necessary.

Volume and specific gravity

The volume varies from 500 to 3000 ml/24 h, average 1500 ml, and depends on the fluid intake and water vapour losses through the skin. *Polyuria* is an increased output of urine, *oliguria* a diminished output, and *anuria* complete suppression of urine. The urine volume must be carefully charted – weighing the patient daily gives a further check of output.

Reaction (acidity)

This is tested by pH indicator paper strip. Urine is normally slightly acid, pH 6. The pH may drop to 4 if metabolism is increased, or in states of acidosis. Ingestion of alkalis and fruits renders the urine alkaline, pH above 7.

Presence of sugar

Glucose is present in the urine in diabetes mellitus, and in patients with a low renal threshold for glucose reabsorption.

Acetone – ketoacids

Ketonuria occurs on severe vomiting, starvation, and diabetic ketosis and coma. It is detected by strip test or tablet.

Protein

Proteinuria is persistent and often heavy in the nephrotic syndrome. It occurs in acute nephritis, hypertensive kidney disease and in chronic renal failure. In urinary tract infections, pus in the urine may cause slight proteinuria but this is not a reliable index of such infection.

Proteinuria may occur in high fever and cardiac failure. In toxaemia of pregnancy there is hypertension, oedema and proteinuria.

Strenuous exercise may cause proteinuria, and in some people it follows prolonged standing, but is absent in a specimen tested after a period of recumbency.

In all these conditions the protein present is albumin, which has a small molecule so that it escapes through the glomeruli.

Bilirubin and urobilinogen

These may be found in the urine in diseases of the liver and biliary tract.

Blood – haematuria

Blood in the urine is called haematuria. If arising from the kidneys the blood will be intimately mixed with the urine. If from the prostate or urethra, blood may only be present at the start of micturition. Painless haematuria most commonly arises in the bladder or prostate, but a renal lesion may be responsible.

Causes

(1) Systemic: blood disorders such as purpura; anticoagulant overdosage.

(2) Renal: acute glomerulonephritis;
renal infarction from arterial thrombosis or embolism;

hypernephroma (carcinoma) – this is painless, there may be a palpable mass;
polycystic disease of the kidneys;
trauma.

(3) Ureteric: stones – usually associated 'renal colic'.

(4) Bladder: papilloma and carcinoma;
schistosomiasis, a parasitic infection.

(5) Prostate: carcinoma.

(6) Urethra: caruncle, and trauma.

A large amount of blood is obvious, lesser quantities give the urine a 'smokey' appearance, or the amount may be so small that microscopical examination is necessary to detect the red cells.

Microscopical examination

This allows the detection of red cells, pus cells (pyuria) and casts. Casts are formed in the renal tubules, and the presence of cellular casts indicates active renal disease.

Specimens for bacteriology

Midstream urine (MSU). A catch specimen in midstream is taken into a sterile wide-mouthed container (preliminary cleansing of the labia in the female with sterile water may be advisable).

The specimen should reach the laboratory within 1 h. The number of colonies of organisms grown, the colony count, is a better index of urinary tract infection than the amount of pus cells present, a colony count of over 100 000/ml urine being significant.

Cytology: an early morning specimen is examined for malignant cells in patients with suspected carcinoma of the urinary tract, especially bladder carcinoma.

(B) BLOOD AND URINE TESTS TO DETERMINE RENAL FUNCTION

Blood urea

The normal blood urea is 2.5–7.5 mmol/l (15–45 mg/dl). The level is raised in renal failure and the rate of rise is more important than the absolute level.

Other routine blood tests include the serum electrolytes sodium, potassium and chloride, acid–base measurements such as pH and bicarbonate, and estimation of calcium and phosphorus.

Clearance tests

The amount of a substance cleared from the plasma by the kidney's filter can be estimated by measuring its plasma concentration, and its urine concentration over a set time. A substance can be injected intravenously for this test, or alternatively one of the substances already present in the plasma can be utilized – urea or creatinine. Thus the creatinine clearance test (estimated on a 6–24 h urine collection) is used clinically as a measure of the glomerular filtration rate and is normally 120 ml/min.

Urine concentration test

The patient is given no fluids after 6 p.m.; the bladder is emptied at 10 p.m. The following morning, the urine specific gravity should be 1022 or higher. The concentrating power of the kidney becomes impaired in disease such as chronic renal failure; the specific gravity being fixed at 1010.

The specific gravity parallels the urea concentration, a healthy kidney being able to produce a urinary area of at least 2 g/100 ml.

(C) X-RAYS

Plain X-ray may show the kidneys, and any opaque stones. In intravenous pyelography (IVP) radio-opaque substance is injected into a forearm vein. It is excreted by the kidneys, demonstrating their size and function, and showing also the renal pelvis, ureters and bladder.

Arteriography

A radio-opaque medium is injected into the aorta near the renal arteries by direct puncture through the lumbar region, or through a catheter inserted from below via the femoral artery. This demonstrates the renal arteries and circulation.

(D) CYSTOSCOPY

This is the examination of the bladder through an instrument passed by the urethra under general anaesthetic. Catheters can be passed into the ureters and a radio-opaque medium allows 'retrograde pyelography'.

(E) RENAL BIOPSY

A specimen of kidney tissue is obtained by a needle inserted through the lumbar region using local anaesthesia. The biopsy is examined by ordinary and electron microscopy. The procedure is contraindicated in bleeding disease and severe uraemia, and carries a risk of causing a renal haematoma.

Common Disorders of the Urinary Tract

(1) URINARY TRACT INFECTION

Cause

Urinary tract infection occurs from bacterial invasion.

(a) *Cystitis* (inflammation of the bladder) from bacterial infection is very common in women, the short urethra in the female allowing entry of bacteria such as *Escherichia coli* (the bowel organism).

(b) *Acute pyelonephritis*
Symptoms and signs
frequency, pain or burning on micturition;

there may be tenderness over the bladder;
pain and tenderness at one or both loins;
rigors and fever;
vomiting is common in children.

(c) *Chronic pyelonephritis*
This may present as recurrent attacks of acute pyelonephritis and loin aches, or there may be symptomless bacteriuria.

(d) *Tuberculosis of the urinary tract*
This was a complication of pulmonary tuberculosis and may still be seen in patients whose drug therapy was non-existent or inadequate, from a lurking focus of infection. The kidneys and bladder are involved; symptoms are those of pyelonephritis and there may be haematuria.

(2) URINARY TRACT STONES (CALCULI)

Symptoms and signs

Renal colic is really ureteric colic from the passage of a stone, which tends to become impacted at the lower end of the ureter.

Pain at the loin, radiating to the groin, building up to maximum severity over about ½ h, then declining only to recur or disappear if the stone is passed into the bladder.

Haematuria may occur.

The stone may eventually pass out through the urethra.

Complications include stasis and infection.

Obstruction may have a back-pressure effect on the kidney, causing hydronephrosis, a dilatation of the renal pelvis, which if infected becomes a pus-containing pyonephrosis.

Renal function becomes impaired.

(3) ACUTE GLOMERULONEPHRITIS (TYPE 1 NEPHRITIS)

This is commonest in children, especially the undernourished, but may occur in adults.

Causes

The commonest cause is an antecedent throat infection with certain strain of haemolytic streptococci. It is an allergic response in both kidneys about 10 days after such infection. Antigen–antibody immune complexes are formed and produce an inflammatory, cellular reaction at the capillaries of the renal glomeruli.

Other disease involving small blood vessels may be causative – anaphylactoid (Henoch–Schönlein) and other purpuras, systemic lupus erythematosus and polyarteritis nodosa.

Symptoms and signs

Oedema, especially of the face, giving a pale, puffy appearance.

Urine is initially diminished in amount.

Haematuria.

Onset is usually abrupt (but there may be history of sore throat).

Malaise.

Shivering, fever.

Aches at the loins.

Blood pressure is slightly raised.

Investigations

Urine contains red cells and casts, is of high specific gravity and may contain protein.

Throat swab and anti-streptolysin O (ASO) titre may confirm antecedent streptococcal infection. The ESR is raised.

Important nursing observations include pulse and temperature chart, blood pressure, daily urine volumes and daily weighing of the patient.

Severe hypertension, persistent proteinuria or rising blood urea occurs in adult acute nephritis; such cases merge into nephrotic syndrome or renal failure.

(4) NEPHROTIC SYNDROME

Causes

Subacute glomerulonephritis (Type 2 nephritis). This is responsible for about 75% of the cases. The cause is unknown but cases may follow an episode of acute glomerulonephritis. It is an immune-complex disease.

Renal vein thrombosis.

Systemic disease affecting the kidneys – amyloid disease, systemic lupus erythematosus, diabetes, malaria, subacute bacterial endocarditis.

Poisons and drugs.

In all these disorders the renal glomeruli have become abnormally porous, leaking out albumin into the urine. The plasma albumin level therefore falls. Albumin in the plasma maintains the osmotic force which attracts water into the circulation. The fall in the plasma albumin results in water passing from the circulation into the tissues, causing oedema. The tendency for the circulating blood volume to fall causes excess aldosterone secretion, with salt and water retention, worsening the tissue oedema.

Symptoms and signs

The first complaint is often ankle swelling, then oedema spreads to the legs, body and face which is pale and puffy.

There may be ascites, and pleural effusion.

There need be no urinary symptoms; perhaps some frothing at micturition due to the albumin in the urine.

Due to the protein loss, which includes some antibodies, resistance is lowered and patients are prone to infection, such as respiratory tract infections.

The course is variable and proteinuria may diminish as diseased nephrons are destroyed but total renal function deteriorates, the patient passing into renal failure.

Investigations

Urine contains 5 g or more albumin per 24 h, but initially is of normal specific gravity. The plasma albumin is low, and the cholesterol high. Blood urea and electrolytes are initially normal.

Renal biopsy may be necessary.

Nursing observations include blood pressure, urine volume and daily weighing of the patient.

(5) RENAL FAILURE

(A) ACUTE RENAL FAILURE

Causes

(1) *Pre-renal* – lack of blood supply to the kidneys:
- (a) haemorrhage – injury, haematemesis;
- (b) fluid loss from vomiting, diarrhoea or severe burns;
- (c) prolonged hypotension from cardiac failure, or septicaemia.

(2) *Renal*:
- (a) some cases of acute nephritis:
- (b) renal cortical necrosis in pregnancy, and the renal damage that may complicate operations in jaundiced patients;
- (c) mis-matched blood transfusion, and following crush injuries causing sludging of blood and nephron damage;
- (d) poisoning by overdose of certain drugs.

(3) *Post-renal*: obstruction in the ureters, bladder or prostate, such as stones, carcinoma, or fibrosis.

Symptoms and signs

There is diminished output of urine.

A history suggestive of renal disease such as polyuria, or anaemia, and the event may have been precipitated by an infection or lowered fluid intake.

Acute uraemia – drowsiness, twitching and vomiting.

(B) CHRONIC RENAL FAILURE – URAEMIA

Chronic renal failure is a disorder of gradual onset, the end result of many chronic diseases of the kidneys. Biochemical evidence of deteriorating renal function, such as a rising blood urea precedes the clinical picture, for symptoms do not appear until 75% of the renal function has been destroyed.

Causes

Chronic glomerulonephritis.

Chronic pyelonephritis.

Hypertensive kidney disease.

Chronic urinary tract obstruction (stones, enlarged prostate).

Less common causes are amyloid disease, systemic lupus erythematosus, gout, diabetes and polycystic disease of the kidneys.

The kidneys are small and scarred. Most of the nephrons have been destroyed, and there is a lack of sufficient numbers to excrete the body's waste products and to control fluid, electrolyte and acid–base balance.

Uraemia, a high blood urea, is the hallmark of renal failure.

Urea is itself non-toxic, but it is the toxic end-products of protein metabolism, plus the systemic effects of the disordered renal function, that cause the symptoms.

Symptoms and signs

Chronic renal failure occurs in middle age, men being more commonly affected (from the effects of hypertension).

Malaise, lack of energy.

Anaemia.

Raised blood pressure.

Polyuria.

Any system may gradually become affected:

DIFFERENTIAL DIAGNOSIS OF PAIN ON URINATION

	Onset	*Course*	*Type of pain*	*Other urinary symptoms*
Acute urethritis	acute	may become chronic	usually burning during urination	frequency; urgency; terminal haematuria may occur
Calculus – bladder or urethral	acute	spontaneous passage may occur	sharp – in glans penis or radiating down penis; burning if infection present	sudden interruption of urinary stream may occur; commonly frequency and urgency; terminal haematuria
Bladder tumours	usually insidious	variable	sharp or burning, most commonly at termination of urination	gross haematuria; with infection – urgency, frequency, nocturia; hesitancy, diminished stream in some
Acute cystitis	acute	usually prompt resolution with therapy	character-istically terminal burning	frequency; nocturia; urge, incontinence; haematuria
Tuberculosis of the urinary tract	insidious	chronic, progressive	usually terminal	frequency; nocturia; haematuria

Associated signs and symptoms	*Other laboratory findings*
urethral discharge; itching or burning in urethra; redness of urethral meatus	Trichomonads, rods, cocci may be found in discharge; bacteria, WBCs in initial portion of urine; cultures may isolate bacteria
often urethral discharge, palpable mass; dull aching or sharp pain increased by movement with bladder calculus	urinalysis – protein, RBCs, WBCs, bacteria; plain film, excretory urograms or cystoscopy for locating calculus
pelvic mass may be palpable; weakness, weight loss, uraemia may develop	anaemia; urinalysis – frequently RBCs WBCs, bacteria; tumour cells may be found on exfoliative cytology; cystogram, cystoscopic examination may be diagnostic
dull suprapubic discomfort; cloudy urine; occasionally tenderness over bladder; pyelonephritis or prostatitis may accompany	leukocytosis; urinalysis – pus cells, bacteria, occasionally RBCs
malaise, fatiguability, fever, night sweats; suprapubic pain; chronic cystitis; thickened epididymis	anaemia; positive tuberculin test; pyuria; urine cultures often positive for *M. tuberculosis;* chest X-ray may show evidence of tuberculosis; X-rays or urograms may show characteristic lesions

DIFFERENTIAL DIAGNOSIS OF HAEMATURIA

	Onset	*Character*	*Pain on urination*	*Course*
Cystitis	usually acute	usually terminal, may be total	dysuria common	usually self-limited; may become chronic
Benign papilloma of the bladder	usually acute	initial, terminal, or total	usually painless	benign, frequently recurrent
Urethritis	usually acute	usually initial, may be terminal	often dysuria	prolonged
Acute glomerulonephritis	acute	total	painless	variable
Chronic glomerulonephritis	insidious	total	painless	usually progressive – eventual renal failure
Trauma to the urinary tract	usually acute	initial, terminal, or total	painless or painful	self-limited or rapidly fatal
Acute pyelonephritis	acute	total	dysuria common	usually self-limited
Nephritis	acute	total	usually painless	usually benign; frequent recurrent attacks with persistence of haematuria

Associated signs and symptoms	*Other laboratory findings*
frequency, low back pain, urgency, lower abdominal pain, lassitude, low-grade fever; sometimes nausea, vomiting, signs of sepsis; cloudy urine; suprapubic tenderness	pyuria; bacteriuria; proteinuria; cystoscopy may show congested mucosa with numerous bleeding points
usually no accompanying signs or symptoms; rarely frequency, urgency, dysuria; occasionally urinary obstruction in females	cystoscopy often shows papilloma; excretory urography may show mass
often urethral discharge, inflammation of urethral mucosa; sometimes frequency, urgency	urine may contain bacteria or WBCs; bacterial culture of urethral discharge positive in 20%
typically, preceding pharyngitis; usually weakness, anorexia; often periorbital oedema; sometimes shortness of breath, hypertension, headache, convulsions; often signs of congestive heart failure; often abdominal pain, nausea, and vomiting; usually scanty urine	often proteinuria; urine sediment shows red blood cells, granular, and epithelial cell casts
sometimes nephrotic syndrome – heavy proteinuria, hypoalbuminaemia, oedema; may progress to signs of renal failure – fatigue, breathlessness, nocturia, nausea, hiccups, pericarditis, pleurisy, insomnia	serum creatinine often elevated; urine sediment may show red blood cells, white blood cells, granular and cellular casts
with renal injury – abdominal pain and tenderness, fulness in loin; with ureteral injury – flank pain, oliguria, fever, azotaemia; with bladder injury – shock and haemorrhage, lower abdominal pain and tenderness, sometimes peritonitis; with urethral injury – pain and extravasation of blood in perineum	intravenous pyelography may be diagnostic
fever, shaking chills, flank pain; often nausea, vomiting; usually tenderness in kidney region	leukocytosis; urine sediment shows many WBCs, WBC casts, RBCs and bacteria; positive urine culture; sometimes positive blood culture
febrile illness or sore throat; hypertension may occur; occasionally joint pain; rarely renal failure, oedema	urine sediment may show red cells, granular, and hyaline casts, proteinuria; renal biopsy shows focal areas of glomerular involvement

(continued overleaf)

DIFFERENTIAL DIAGNOSIS OF HAEMATURIA (cont'd)

	Onset	*Character*	*Pain on urination*	*Course*
Renal calculi	usually acute	total	painful when renal colic present	usually self-limited, often recurrent
Carcinoma of the bladder	usually insidious	frequently terminal	painless unless passage of clots causes obstruction	progressive

Associated signs and symptoms	*Other laboratory findings*
renal colic common; often frequency, vomiting; sometimes tachycardia, hypotension, often tenderness in renal area	X-rays may demonstrate stones; urine sediment may show bacteria or crystals; sometimes abnormal serum calcium, phosphorus, uric acid, alkaline phosphatase
often associated urinary tract infection; uraemia, anaemia, weight loss in advanced cases; pelvic mass may be palpable	cystogram may demonstrate urethral obstruction, filling defect of bladder or flattening of bladder wall; cystoscopy will visualize tumour

DIFFERENTIAL DIAGNOSIS OF OLIGURIA AND ANURIA

	Oliguria and/ or anuria	*Onset*	*Course*
Dehydration	oliguria more common	insidious or acute	reversible with correction of dehydration
Congestive heart failure	usually oliguria, rarely anuria	acute or insidious	reversible with correction of CHF
Acute glomerulonephritis	oliguria more common	acute	usually recovery in 1–2 weeks, occasionally irreversible renal failure
Acute toxaemia of pregnancy	oliguria in severe pre-eclampsia, anuria in eclampsia	insidious or acute	usually recovery with termination of pregnancy
Multiple myeloma	anuria or oliguria	acute onset	usually fatal outcome
Renal failure – end-stage chronic renal disease	oliguria progressing to anuria	insidious	fatal progression unless dialysis or transplant

Associated signs and symptoms	*Other laboratory findings*
thirst, fever; lassitude; tachycardia, postural hypotension common; dryness of tongue and lips, loss of skin tone typical	often ECG abnormalities; serum hypertonicity, elevated serum sodium; usually haemoconcentration; high urine specific gravity, low urine sodium and chloride, normal urine sediment
anorexia, nausea, vomiting common; often dyspnoea, orthopnoea, haemoptysis; sometimes pulmonary rales and oedema; often gallop rhythms, cardiomegaly, tachycardia; distended neck veins; hepatomegaly, peripheral oedema	characteristic chest X-ray; urine shows high specific gravity, high urea, low sodium, often proteinuria and microscopic haematuria
preceding pharyngitis frequent; malaise, nausea, headache, anorexia common; often facial oedema; 'smokey' brown urine typical; usually mild hypertension; signs of CHF in some; often pain in loins or abdomen	throat cultures may be positive for streptococcus; usually elevated ASLO titre, diminished globulin; proteinuria common; urine sediment; many RBCs and WBCs; small number of renal tubular cells; granular, RBC and hyaline casts
oedema, weight gain, hypertension typical in pre-eclampsia; convulsion, coma in eclampsia; visual disturbances may occur; sometimes nausea, vomiting; cardiac failure may develop	often haemoconcentration, hyperuricaemia; typically proteinuria; urine sediment: a few RBCs, granular or hyaline casts
weakness, anorexia, weight loss, back pain common; sometimes peripheral neuropathies; often bony lesions; macroglossia	often rouleaux formation, elevated ESR; usually hypercalcaemia, hyperuricaemia, hyperproteinuria; Bence Jones proteinuria may be present; normal urine sediment; osteolytic bone lesions on X-ray; myeloma cells in bone marrow
dry mouth, anorexia, vomiting, diarrhoea; sometimes pruritus, yellow complexion; heart failure in some; often hypertension, pericarditis, pericardial friction rub; sometimes insomnia, convulsions; epistaxis, gastrointestinal haemorrhage may occur	usually normochromic, normocytic anaemia; hyponatraemia, hyperkalaemia, acidosis, hypocalcaemia, hyperphosphataemia, hypermagnesaemia, hyperuricaemia may be present; urine sediment: proteinuria, casts; bony changes on X-ray

Cardiovascular system: hypertension, pulmonary oedema, arrhythmias from high potassium, terminal pericarditis.

Respiratory: deep sighing, breathing of acidosis (blowing off CO_2).

Alimentary: anorexia, nausea, vomiting, hiccups, dry tongue and stomatitis, later diarrhoea which may become bloody.

Haemopoietic: anaemia and bleeding tendency.

Nervous system: convulsions, coma, peripheral neuropathy.

Skin: brown, yellow pigmentation, pruritus, purpura.

Skeletal: bones may be decalcified (osteomalacia) calcium deposited in tissues, or tetany may occur from a low blood calcium.

Patients may tolerate mild symptoms for many years. Deterioration may be provoked by infection or inadequate fluid intake.

Investigations

The urine is of large volume, fixed specific gravity around 1010 and poor urea content (less than 1 g/l). Proteinuria may be present. A midstream specimen should be cultured. Frequent weighing of the patient is a guide to fluid balance.

Straight X-ray shows small kidneys. IVP may be performed, but the kidneys may be unable to concentrate the medium adequately for visualization.

The blood urea [normal 2.5–7.5 mmol/l (15–45 mg/dl)] is raised: a level of 20–30 mmol/l (120–180 mg/dl) may be tolerated for years, and a sudden rise is more significant than the absolute level. The blood creatinine (another protein metabolite) is raised and its level is independent of protein in the diet. The creatinine clearance test is a guide to the glomerular filtration rate, roughly parallels residual renal function, and may drop to 10% of normal or even less in the terminal stage. The serum sodium, potassium and degree of acidosis (low pH or bicarbonate) are measured.

Chapter 8

The Central and Peripheral Nervous System

Apart from cerebrovascular disease or 'strokes', there are few diseases of the central nervous system (CNS) that are common. Strokes are a major cause of death – at least 10% of all deaths (the third commonest cause in Western countries) – but other CNS and neurological disorders cause relatively few deaths – less than 1%. Migraine, epilepsy, head injury, tumour, paralysis agitans, vertigo and multiple sclerosis are the main disorders of this system leading to either initial consultation or hospital admission – and they occur, in incidence, in that order of frequency in the population.

Diagnosis of disorder will depend on symptoms, history, observation of the patient and examination of:

(A) central and peripheral nervous system reflexes,
(B) retina by ophthalmoscopy,
(C) X-rays – straight, scan and contrast,
(D) lumbar puncture,
(E) electroencephalography,
(F) electromyography.

Common symptoms of disorder will be:

(1) loss of muscular function,
(2) loss of consciousness,
(3) headache,
(4) neuralgia,
(5) dizziness and disorientation,
(6) nausea and vomiting.

(A) THE NERVOUS SYSTEM REFLEXES

The spinal reflex arc consists of the sensory fibres which receive information from the periphery and pass it via the posterior root into the spinal cord, where a connector neurone passes it to the anterior horn cells, from which the stimulus passes out to cause muscular contraction.

Damage to the reflex arc at any part of its course results in loss of a 'deep' (or tendon) reflex such as the knee jerk, normally produced by contraction of the quadriceps muscle following the sensory stimulus of a tap on the patella tendon with the tendon hammer.

The activity of the reflex arc and its lower motor neurone fibres is influenced by the upper motor neurone.

A lower motor neurone lesion is characterized by muscle weakness or flaccid paralysis followed by wasting, and loss of the tendon reflexes. Groups of muscles in a limb rather than the whole limb are involved.

An upper motor neurone lesion is characterized by muscular weakness, that is paralysis, tending to affect the whole of one or more limbs. There is an increase in muscle tone causing rigidity or spasticity, and exaggerated tendon reflexes, e.g. excessively brisk knee and ankle jerks; these may keep jerking after the stimulus is withdrawn, the phenomenon called clonus. There may also be abnormality of 'superficial' reflexes with an 'extensor plantar response' (Babinski's sign) where the big toe goes upwards and the other toes fan outwards and upwards when the lateral border of the sole of the foot is stroked, instead of the normal downward 'flexor' movement. An upper motor neurone lesion is also associated with absent abdominal reflexes – that is stroking the skin of the abdomen fails to elicit the normal contraction of the muscles of the abdominal wall.

An upper motor neurone lesion causes a hemiplegia – a paralysis of one side of the body including the lower half of the face, the arm, and the leg. (Classically caused by a stroke – haemorrhage or ischaemia – affecting the internal capsule containing the pyramidal tract.) Paralysis of both legs is called paraplegia.

A more extensive lesion in the brain may involve fibres radiating from the optic nerves and tracts, causing loss of the field of vision. Any lesion of the pyramidal tract may also involve speech fibres, causing expressive dysphasia – difficulty in finding the word. Larger lesions affecting the hearing area or its fibres cause receptive language difficulties, and the patient is incoherent and confused.

Small areas of destruction of the cerebral cortex may cause apraxia, a disorder of the motor act – thus the patient may have normal power and be able to hold a box of matches, but he is incapable of striking a light; similarly, agnosia is a disorder of sensory appreciation – crude sensation such as pain and touch is retained, but the patient is unable to state the nature of an object placed in his hand.

Apart from the sensations such as pain, temperature and touch reaching consciousness, the sensory fibres convey information on muscle tone and balance, proprioception, and disturbance results in ataxia and inco-ordination of muscular movement. Ataxia may result from destruction of the posterior columns of the spinal cord, resulting in a reeling or drunken gait. Inco-ordination of movement also occurs in lesions of the cerebellum or its connections in the brain stem as in multiple sclerosis, so that the patient 'overshoots the mark' when trying to grasp an object and has a tremor, called intention tremor, as he is about to reach it. Nystagmus can be regarded as an intention tremor of the eyes when fixing on an object, due to inco-ordination of the external ocular muscles.

(B) EXAMINATION OF THE RETINA (OPTIC FUNDUS) WITH THE OPHTHALMOSCOPE

Papilloedema may be seen in raised intracranial pressure and hypertension. In hypertension, arteriosclerosis and diabetes, retinal vessel changes and haemorrhages may be visible. In subarachnoid haemorrhage there may be a small pool of blood at the retina.

(C) X-RAYS, STRAIGHT, SCAN AND CONTRAST

(i) STRAIGHT X-RAYS

The skull may be invaded, or show evidence of raised intracranial pressure, in cerebral tumour, but such changes are late. A calcified pineal gland may show a shift from its normal central position due to a space-occupying lesion. Chest X-ray should always be carried out, for a brain tumour may be a secondary from bronchogenic carcinoma.

(ii) COMPUTERIZED AXIAL TOMOGRAPHY

Also known as CAT scan. This form of X-ray has revolutionized diagnosis in neurology; it gives an anatomical picture of the brain, and soft tissues and abnormalities such as tumours and haemorrhage can be recognized. It is a 'non-invasive' investigation causing no discomfort to the patient.

(iii) RADIOISOTOPE BRAIN SCANNING

Certain radioactive isotopes are selectively taken up by brain tumours which can be detected by a counter scan or 'scanner' over the skull.

(iv) CEREBRAL ANGIOGRAPHY (ARTERIOGRAPHY)

This is the injection of a dye, opaque to X-rays, into a blood vessel, usually a large artery such as the carotid. Its branches inside the skull can be seen on X-ray using a cinematograph technique. Aneurysms and vascular abnormalities may be identified.

(v) MYELOGRAPHY

Here an iodine-containing substance, opaque to X-rays, is

injected at lumbar puncture to show the presence of a spinal cord blockage.

(D) ELECTROENCEPHALOGRAPHY (EEG)

A series of recordings of the electrical activity of the brain using electrodes attached to the head. The test indicates localized abnormality of brain function over areas of softening or tumour and may show local or general abnormalities of electrical activity characteristic of the several types of epilepsy.

(E) LUMBAR PUNCTURE

A specimen of cerebrospinal fluid (CSF) is obtained by inserting a needle, under local anaesthesia, into the subarachnoid space below the level where the spinal cord ends (which is opposite the lower border of the first lumbar vertebrae). The needle is usually inserted between the 3rd–4th or 4th–5th lumbar vertebrae with the patient held curled-up in the left lateral position. Lumbar puncture should not generally be carried out if there is papilloedema, for raised intracranial pressure may cause downward 'coning' of the brain against the skull if fluid is taken off from below.

At lumbar puncture, the CSF pressure is measured with a manometer, normal is 50–150 mm of fluid, and there should be a free rise and fall on pressing and releasing each jugular vein in turn, excluding any blockage. Normal CSF is crystal clear, contains virtually no cells and has a protein content of less than 0.4 g/l (40 mg/dl). White cells may be increased in inflammatory conditions and bacteriological culture will confirm infections. The CSF is heavily blood-stained in subarachnoid haemorrhage and sometimes after intracerebral haemorrhage. Abnormalities in the CSF protein are fractionated chemically; they occur in neurosyphilis, multiple sclerosis and acute ascending polyneuritis.

(F) NERVE CONDUCTION STUDIES AND ELECTROMYOGRAPHY

These electrical techniques may define peripheral nerve

changes and allow differentiation of nerve and muscle disease.

Common Disorders of the Central and Peripheral Nervous System

(1) CEREBROVASCULAR DISEASE

In elderly people the cerebral arteries are very liable to be affected by arteriosclerosis usually as part of more widespread arterial involvement. Arteriosclerosis is a degenerative change of the lining membrane of the artery associated with patchy fatty deposits with tendency to thrombosis and aggregation of platelets on the roughened surface.

The arteriosclerotic change has two effects – it narrows the arterial lumen (which may become completely obstructed), and the plaque is a source of emboli which may impact in a distal, smaller artery, causing ischaemia or infarction at a distance from the main vessel.

STROKE, CEREBROVASCULAR ACCIDENT, APOPLEXY

A stroke – a cerebrovascular accident – is an abrupt loss of function of some part of the brain due to an arterial lesion.

The common stroke of the elderly results in hemiplegia, a branch of the middle cerebral artery serving the internal capsule may have been affected by thrombosis, or haemorrhage, or an embolism may have travelled from the heart. Haemorrhage is more catastrophic with destruction of brain tissue and often death. The differentiation of thrombosis and haemorrhage may be impossible.

Many strokes are also due to arterial disease affecting the internal carotid artery in the neck, narrowing its lumen and being a source of emboli.

Many major strokes are preceded by transient ischaemic attacks with impairment of function lasting less than an hour. These little strokes are often due to small emboli from an internal carotid artery thrombosis.

(a) Minor strokes

Symptoms and signs

Transient weakness of the arm and leg.

Blindness affecting the eye on the same side as the lesion.

A murmur ('bruit') may be heard with the stethoscope over the narrowed internal arotid artery.

Dizziness.

Cranial nerve palsies and sometimes momentary loss of consciousness with a 'drop attack'.

Recurrent episodes contribute to intellectual deterioration.

(b) Major strokes

Symptoms and signs

Weakness, or paralysis of one side of the body – hemiplegia.

Onset is generally sudden.

Frontal headache.

Dysphasia may occur from involvement of the speech centre.

Disturbance of cerebration, or the patient may be found unconscious.

Deepening coma with no response to commands or to painful stimuli.

Stertorous or periodic breathing of Cheyne–Stokes type.

Pulse slow but full.

Incontinence of urine.

In severe cases, all four limbs may be flaccid, both plantar responses extensor and deterioration may be rapid with death in hours or a day or two.

In the majority of strokes, however, the lesion is an ischaemic rather than a haemorrhagic one, and consciousness is quickly regained or improves over hours or a few days. The paralysis affects the lower half of the face, the arm and the leg, but the limbs may be initially flaccid and remain so, or develop the classical spasticity of the upper motor neurone lesion, with extensor plantar response. Difficulty in swallowing and articulation is usually transient.

A hemiplegia may be accompanied by loss of sensation on the paralysed side, and if the lesion is more extensive, involvement of the optic radiation causes loss of one half of the visual field – thus a lesion in the left internal capsule can cause right hemiplegia, dysphasia, right hemi-anaesthesia, and right hemianopia – the patient may not be aware of objects on the right side of his body and may ignore that side.

There is usually little difficulty in distinguishing a stroke from other neurological conditions – a stroke is a vascular occlusion or haemorrhage and of sudden onset, distinct from the gradual onset of symptoms from a cerebral tumour.

Regular observations – of level of consciousness, pulse, blood pressure, respiration, temperature, fluid intake and urine output – should be made. Deterioration of consciousness, a slowing pulse and rising blood pressure suggest rising intracranial pressure or cerebral destruction. Hyperpyrexia, with pinpoint pupils, may occur in haemorrhage.

(2) INTRACRANIAL HAEMORRHAGE

The forms of brain haemorrhage are:

(i) Intracerebral haemorrhage

As in 'Stroke' above.

(ii) Subarachnoid haemorrhage

Due to rupture of a small aneurysm of one of the arteries at the base of the brain. The aneurysm forms as a result of a developmental defect in the vessel wall, and it manifests in adult life.

Symptoms and signs

Commonest in young and middle-aged adults.

Warning headache or neckache.

Days later the patient suffers severe and often agonizing headache and neckache with neck stiffness.

Sudden loss of consciousness with deep coma and flaccid weakness of all limbs.

Diagnosis is confirmed by lumbar puncture which reveals heavily blood-stained cerebrospinal fluid.

CAT scan shows the site of haemorrhage and may reveal the aneurysm causing it.

Angiography subsequently allows detailed assessment of the aneurysm and blood vessels.

(iii) Extradural haemorrhage

This follows a head injury, usually with fracture of the temporal bone of the skull, and is due to rupture of the middle meningeal artery.

The patient may have been transiently stunned, then there is a 'lucid interval', and then deepening coma from the pressure effects of the bleeding displacing the brain – there may be a dilated pupil.

CAT scanning and surgical aspiration of the haemorrhage are indicated.

(iv) Subdural haemorrhage

A more slowly developing collection of blood from ruptured veins in the subdural space.

It occurs in birth injury, and also in the elderly, possibly because of some shrinkage of brain substance and weakening of the walls of the veins, which rupture after relatively trivial injury.

A history of injury to the head, which may have been forgotten, and the skull may or may not have been fractured.

Days or weeks later there is disturbance of consciousness or lateralizing signs, and the condition may be mistaken for a stroke. The subdural haemorrhage is one form of 'space-occupying-lesion' and the treatment is surgical.

(3) SPACE-OCCUPYING LESIONS OF THE BRAIN

These are haematomas, cerebral tumours or abscesses.

Symptoms and signs

(i) Local effects

By destroying the brain substance, the lesion may cause complaints such as difficulty in moving part of a limb, or disorder of the motor act (apraxia).

Speech disturbance, transient deafness or defective sense of smell.

The personality may change with behaviour disorders, e.g. inappropriate urination.

There may be focal fits related to disturbance in electrical function.

(ii) Displacement effects

A nerve may be displaced and stretched – thus there may be paralysis of the sixth cranial nerve with resultant orbital muscle weakness and double vision (diplopia)

A tumour such as the 'acoustic neuroma' not only causes deafness and ataxia (disturbance of gait) but also causes loss of the corneal reflex from stretching of the fifth and seventh cranial nerves.

(iii) Raised intracranial pressure

Diffuse pressure effects on brain metabolism and disturbance of the normal circulation of the cerebrospinal fluid.

Headache.

Vomiting.

Drowsiness.

Slowing of the pulse and of the respiratory rate.

Papilloedema.

Confirming the presence of space-occupying lesion

Skull X-ray may show a displacement of the pineal gland from the midline should the gland be calcified as it often is in middle age; some tumours are calcified.

Raised intracranial pressure may cause erosion of the bone near the pituitary fossa – which can itself be enlarged in pituitary tumour.

Chest X-ray may show a primary tumour in the lung.

CAT scanning shows the site and often the nature of the lesion.

Isotope scanning and EEG may be useful in confirmation.

(4) INFECTIONS OF THE CENTRAL NERVOUS SYSTEM

(i) MENINGITIS

An acute inflammation of the meninges, usually bacterial, spread having occurred from a septic process penetrating the skull following injury or operation, or via the bloodstream from a distant focus, e.g., the throat.

Symptoms and signs

Meningococcal meningitis is commonest in young people, especially in closed communities which may allow spread of infection from throat or nasal secretions.

Onset is usually acute with headache, neckache and neck stiffness.

Inability to straighten the knee when the hip is flexed (Kernig's sign) – due to the inflamed meninges irritating the nerve roots.

Clouding of consciousness.

Diagnosis is confirmed by lumbar puncture. The cerebrospinal fluid may be under raised pressure, is cloudy due to pus cells in the bacterial cases and the organisms can be cultured from it.

(ii) ENCEPHALITIS AND ENCEPHALOMYELITIS

The enteroviruses, which include the poliomyelitis, Echo and Coxsackie viruses, spread in the bloodstream to reach the nervous system and cause an encephalitis, an inflammation of the brain cells, or in the case of poliomyelitis the virus tends to localize at the anterior horn cells of the spinal cord.

The virus of herpes simplex, which normally cause only 'cold sores' at the mouth, can at times cause a severe encephalitis; similar viruses are responsible for epidemics of encephalitis occurring in the tropics and the Far East.

The childhood fevers – measles, mumps, rubella (German measles) and chickenpox – may be accompanied or followed by virus invasion of the nervous system resulting in encephalitis or encephalomyelitis and mild meningitis. Encephalomyelitis may also follow glandular fever (infectious mononucleosis), and vaccination against measles and smallpox.

Encephalomyelitis is characterized by patchy demyelination of the insulating and nutritive myelin sheath that surrounds the nerve fibres in the brain and spinal cord. Demyelination may also involve the peripheral nerves.

Symptoms and signs

Often mild, and the illness transient.

In severe cases there is fever, disturbance of cerebration with intellectual disturbance, emotional upset and clouding of consciousness. The patient resents interference.

Sleep rhythm may be upset.

Headache.

Vomiting.

Neck stiffness.

Cranial nerve palsies and additional motor or sensory impairment from peripheral nerve involvement.

At lumbar puncture, the CSF may be normal or show increased cells or protein.

Blood may show a rising virus antibody titre.

Virus may be cultured from the stools, in which enteroviruses survive for up to 24 h at room temperature.

The EEG may show diffuse electrical disturbance of the brain.

(iii) RABIES

Rabies is a virus infection which results in a form of encephalitis, usually fatal. The virus is transmitted to humans through bites from infected animals, especially dogs, but bats are also carriers. If a person is bitten, he must be given an immediate course of anti-rabies vaccination, otherwise the virus passes up the nerves to reach the brain.

Symptoms include

Muscular stiffness.

Convulsions.

Paralysis of swallowing.

Coma and death.

(iv) POLIOMYELITIS

This is increasingly rare due to effective vaccination. The poliomyelitis virus is of the enterovirus group, colonizing in the intestinal tract and excreted in the faeces. Thus infection is still common in underdeveloped countries with poor hygiene and primitive sanitation. The virus spreads to the CNS, affecting mainly the anterior horn cells of the spinal cord, though the brain stem may also be involved.

Symptoms and signs

Initial febrile illness, often with signs of meningeal irritation.

Followed by paralysis of sudden onset, usually affecting one leg or arm.

If the phrenic nerve supplying the diaphragm, and the nerves to the intercostal muscles, are involved, respiration becomes impossible.

Involvement of cranial nerves results in difficulty in speaking and swallowing, and the respiratory centre in the medulla can also be affected.

(v) HERPES ZOSTER (SHINGLES)

This is a virus infection of the posterior (sensory) nerve root ganglia. The virus is the same as that causing chickenpox in children. Herpes zoster is commonest in the middle-aged and elderly, the virus possibly lying dormant in the nervous system. The condition may only appear if the patient is debilitated, or it may accompany an irritative lesion such as a tumour near the nerve root.

Symptoms and signs

'Herpes' describes the herpetic or vesicular eruption, and 'zoster' means its band-like distribution along the line of a nerve, often an intercostal nerve.

A painful, itchy vesicular rash commonly at the trunk, but any nerve can be involved.

The ophthalmic division of the fifth (trigeminal) cranial nerve may be affected with typical rash on one half of the forehead, and painful redness of the eye.

(vi) TETANUS (LOCKJAW)

The spores of the bacillus *Clostridium tetani* causing tetanus are found in manure, soil and dust. Like the gas gangrene organisms, the tetanus bacilli grow best where the oxygen supply is poor, and infection follows contamination of deep punctures and wounds.

Tetanus is due to a toxin produced by the bacilli growing in a wound. This toxin travels up the peripheral nerves to reach the CNS.

(vii) BOTULISM

Botulism is a form of food poisoning due to a bacterial toxin which blocks the release of acetylcholine at nerve endings, causing widespread paralysis. The spores of the bacillus producing the toxin (*Clostridium botulinum*), like those of tetanus, are found in soil and faeces. They multiply in anaerobic conditions as in canned foods or home-bottled fruit which has been inadequately sterilized. The spores themselves resist boiling but the toxin is easily destroyed by cooking.

Symptoms and signs

Some vomiting but seldom pain or diarrhoea.

The absorbed toxin paralyses nerve endings.

Difficulty in talking and swallowing.

Double vision and giddiness.

Paralysis extends to the trunk and limbs and death may follow from respiratory failure.

(5) MULTIPLE SCLEROSIS (DISSEMINATED SCLEROSIS)

Multiple sclerosis is a chronic disease of the nervous system, almost always arising before the age of 40. It is characterized by remissions and relapses and by the presence of multiple patches of sclerosis scattered throughout the brain and the spinal cord.

Cause

The cause is unknown. The disease affects 1 in 2000 of the population of the UK and the USA, is commonest in temperate northern climates, rare in the tropics and South Africa, and unknown in China and Japan. Multiple sclerosis is a demyelinating disease – the myelin sheath, which protects and nourishes the nerve fibre (just as insulation protects an electric cable) is destroyed by some unknown agent. Conduction in the underlying nerve fibres is at first only temporarily affected, and early changes may be reversible, but later, plaques of scar tissue are formed, destroying the nerve fibres.

The demyelination bears some resemblance to lesions in encephalomyelitis and a virus cause has been suggested, or an infective agent, aggravated by stress, injury, infection or in the puerperium. Multiple sclerosis may be a disturbance of immunity resulting in change in the fatty acids of the myelin sheaths.

Symptoms and signs

These are disseminated – in time and in place.

The presenting sign is often a transient weakness of arm or leg or a blurring of vision which clears up.

Months or years later there are more permanent signs.

The pyramidal tracts are commonly involved causing spastic weakness, becoming fairly symmetrical in both legs.

Sensory changes are slight.

There is often disturbance of bladder function such as urgency of micturition, incontinence, or retention.

Cranial nerve involvement includes the optic nerve causing the visual disturbance and sometimes pallor of the optic disc seen with the ophthalmoscope.

The cerebellum and its connections may be involved, causing disorder of muscle balance and control and ataxia.

There is a fine tremor of the fingers, more marked on movement (intention tremor) and brought out by the 'finger–nose' test, as the patient, starting with hand outstretched, brings in the index finger to touch the tip of the nose.

There is inability to perform rapid to-and-fro movements of the hands.

A similar disturbance of the ocular muscles causes the fine tremor of the eyes, called nystagmus, when attempt is made to fix the gaze on an object held in front.

The voice may have a peculiar staccato quality.

There may be acute exacerbations of symptoms, settling in early cases and followed by months or even years of remission.

In severe cases there is gradual deterioration over the years, the patient becoming paraplegic (paralysed in both legs) and incontinent, unable to get out of bed without help, and prone to urinary and chest infections and to pressure sores.

Further investigations

Lumbar puncture. In half the cases of multiple sclerosis, the cerebrospinal fluid shows an increase in the gammaglobulin fraction of the protein.

Apart from routine ones such as urine testing, blood count and chest X-ray, further investigations are seldom required, but myelography may be indicated in the occasional patient with purely pyramidal tract signs, to exclude a tumour or other lesion causing compression of the spinal cord.

(6) SYNCOPE

This is transient loss of consciousness due to inadequate cerebral blood flow.

(i) FAINT (VASOVAGAL ATTACK)

Occurs in healthy people, usually the young, and is a feeling of light-headedness which is followed by collapse – the person has some warning of an impending faint.

Causes

Precipitating factors may be psychogenic – emotion, an unpleasant sight, fear of an injection, or the presence of severe pain (cardiac pain, renal 'colic'). These result in vagal stimulation with lowered peripheral resistance and pooling of blood, causing reduced venous return and cardiac output. The heart is also slowed. Prolonged standing in the erect posture in a hot climate also causes venous pooling, with the same result.

Symptoms and signs

Pallor.

Sweating.

Feeling of sickness and swimming in the head.

Loss of consciousness and collapse.

The pulse is slow and the blood pressure lowered, but as soon as the person is flat, the cerebral circulation improves and consciousness returns in a few seconds.

(ii) CARDIAC SYNCOPE

This occurs in the older age groups, and usually there is a known history of heart disease. Fainting occurs on effort in patients whose hearts cannot meet the demand for blood created by exercise, and there is temporary cerebral anoxia – this may occur in aortic stenosis or mitral stenosis.

Stokes–Adams attacks are sudden episodes of cerebral anoxia following heart block, with return of consciousness and facial flushing when the ventricle restarts. The onset of atrial fibrillation or other arrhythmia may also cause temporary cerebral ischaemia.

Sino-atrial disease ('sick-sinus syndrome') associated with rhythm disturbance and sinus arrest, may have similar effects in the elderly.

Carotid-sinus syncope is due to pressure of a tight collar stimulating the carotid sinus nerves with resultant reflex hypotension.

Cough syncope ('cough drop') occurs when a patient, frequently a chronic bronchitic, coughs so much that he impedes the venous return to the heart, resulting in collapse.

(7) EPILEPSY

A group of conditions characterized by recurrent attacks of disordered brain function called seizures or fits. Fits are of sudden onset and each is usually short in duration, lasting only a matter of minutes.

Cause

Epilepsy results from disordered electrical activity of the brain. The fit is due to an abnormal electrical focus firing off a discharge with resultant disturbance of cerebration and usually loss of consciousness.

TYPES OF EPILEPSY

Symptomatic epilepsy

Due to some definable irritant focus, the epilepsy is a symptom of the underlying disorder. Thus epilepsy may follow damage to the brain at birth, or head injury, or indicate the presence of a space-occupying lesion such as tumour, abscess or haematoma, or result from a scar of the brain after a stroke.

Idiopathic epilepsy

In the vast majority of cases of epilepsy, no reason for the electrical instability can be discovered – 80% of the patients belong to this group.

The incidence of known epilepsy is 5 per 1000 of the population but the condition may go unrecognized, and many people have an epileptic attack at some time during their lives. There is a familial tendency, the incidence of epilepsy in the children being slightly higher if one parent is affected, and considerably higher if both parents have known epilepsy.

Factors precipitating an attack include fatigue and stress, over-hydration, anoxia and metabolic causes such as uraemia, hypoglycaemia and hypocalcaemia. Fits also occur in severe toxaemia of pregnancy – eclampsia. A flickering television screen may provoke a fit due to the stroboscopic effect. More often, no precipitating cause can be recognized.

PETIT MAL — MINOR EPILEPSY

Symptoms and signs

Arises in children or adolescents and never starts in adult life.

A transitory interruption of consciousness, without any convulsive element. The patient simply stops what he is doing or saying and may stare vacantly into space for a few seconds before resuming his previous activity. He seldom, if ever, falls, and he has no realization that anything abnormal has occurred.

Attacks may occur once every few weeks or months, or there may be several in one day.

Diagnosis should be possible from a description of the attacks, and can be confirmed by the electroencephalogram, which shows a characteristic spike-and-wave pattern.

GRAND MAL — MAJOR EPILEPSY

This commonly begins between the ages of 7 and 17. Attacks starting in adult life should raise the suspicion of a brain lesion such as a tumour. The fit is almost always of sudden onset and has three stages:

The major fit

Tonic stage

The patient may cry out, consciousness is suddenly lost and he falls to the ground.

All the muscles are in rigid spasm, so he falls heavily and may injure himself.

The limbs are extended, the jaw clenched and the tongue may be bitten.

Respiration ceases, resulting in cyanosis. (This tonic stage lasts for about half a minute.)

Clonic stage

Muscle twitching often starts at the fingers or around the mouth, then the limb muscles contract and relax, causing jerking movements.

These movements spread, becoming violent and convulsive, the arms and legs thrashing about with risk of further injury, but breathing is resumed.

The muscle jerkings involve the jaw and mouth, so the tongue may be bitten again and with foaming of the saliva the patient froths at the mouth.

There may be incontinence of urine. (This stage lasts for 1–3 min after which the movements gradually cease.)

Somnolent stage

The patient now passes into a deep sleep or coma, remaining unrousable for a few minutes or up to an hour.

During this, and the clonic stage, the pupils and reflexes may be abnormal with extensor plantar responses.

The patient may subsequently feel drowsy and sometimes complains of headache.

Amnesia.

Occasionally there is a period of post-epileptic automatism during which the patient may carry out some action of which he is unaware.

Status epilepticus
The occurrence of a series of major fits, the patient passing from one fit to another without regaining consciousness. The patient may become hyperpyrexial, and the periods of anoxia may precipitate brain damage.

Further investigations in grand mal

It is essential to obtain an eye-witness account of the fit and usually this allows diagnosis.

Electroencephalography
The EEG shows an electrical abnormality of the brain which may be of localizing value, or it may be generalized.

Most cases of epilepsy are idiopathic, but the fact that the condition may be a symptom of an underlying lesion such as a tumour should be borne in mind, especially where fits start in adult life.

A full clinical examination, including ophthalmoscopy and urine testing, blood count and blood sugar estimations, and X-rays of chest and skull are necessary but if a space-occupying lesion is suspected CAT scan is indicated. Lumbar puncture need not be done routinely but a raised CSF protein would heighten a suspicion of tumour.

(8) HEADACHE

Headache is a common symptom which generally has no serious cause, but it can be associated with organic disorder. The brain itself is insensitive to pain but intracranial structures such as the arteries and meninges are pain-sensitive. Spasm of the cervical muscles also results in pain.

Causes of headache

(i) Vascular

The headache accompanying fever is probably due to dilatation of intracranial arteries. Migraine headache (see below) is due to dilatation of extracranial arteries in the external carotid system. The same mechanism explains the headache that may occur with internal carotid artery thrombosis.

Headache may occur in cerebral haemorrhage before consciousness is lost – in subarachnoid haemorrhage there is severe occipital headache and neck stiffness, and there may have been a prolonged neck-ache from leakage of the aneurysm aneurysm a few days earlier.

Temporal (cranial) arteritis is one of the connective tissue autoimmune diseases, and is an inflammation of the arteries of the skull, with headache and tenderness at the temple, usually unilaterally. The condition may involve the retinal arteries, leading to blindness, and it is commonest in elderly men. The ESR is raised.

(ii) Tumour and raised intracranial pressure

Tumour may cause headache which is dull in character, rarely severe and tends to occur early in the day.

Though raised intracranial pressure from any cause, can produce a generalized headache, its intensity need not be related to the height of the pressure.

(iii) Inflammation and irritation

Meningitis and encephalitis can cause severe headache. There is also neck-ache and neck stiffness. Occipital headache and neck stiffness occurs also in subarachnoid haemorrhage.

Sinusitis – stuffy, headachy feelings and tenderness over the affected part.

Eye causes – 'eye strain' from refractive errors may cause evening headaches. Glaucoma – raised intraocular pressure, with risk of loss of vision, and often accompanying vomiting – is a cause of headache in the elderly.

(iv) Cervical spondylosis – 'tension' headache

This is a form of arthritis affecting the cervical spine. There is associated muscle spasm with pain and tenderness at the neck, often spreading to cause a generalized headache. Symptoms are worse in tense, anxious patients, their state probably contributing to increased muscle tension – 'tension' headache.

(v) Depression

Depression and psychogenic factors lie behind many chronic or recurrent headaches, muscle tension making the symptoms worse.

(vi) Migraine

Migraine is recurrent attacks of headache, often in bouts for a week or two, then there may be freedom for months. Migraine begins in adolescence, often there is a family history and attacks tend to be less severe after middle age. Sufferers are often of a tense, worrying personality. Attacks may occur premenstrually, possibly due to fluid retention.

Symptoms and signs

The 'aura' – due to spasm of intracranial arteries – may present as 'flashing lights' or visual upset, minutes or even some hours before the next stage.

Headache is often localized to the region of the superficial temporal artery on one part of the head, and it is usually the same part that is involved in each attack.

The headache may be so severe that the patient has to lie down in a dark room to gain relief.

Occasionally there is weakness of a limb or one side of the body (hemiplegic migraine).

Nausea and vomiting – may complicate or follow the headache.

(9) PARALYSIS AGITANS

A chronic and progressive disease due to degenerative changes in the basal ganglia of the brain; it is a common condition in the middle-aged and elderly.

Cause

In all types there are degenerative changes in the basal ganglia, the nuclei at the base of the brain or their connections, which form part of the extrapyramidal system concerned in normal muscle tone. It is associated with depletion of a substance called dopamine, a neurological chemical transmitter. Dopamine regulates the function of the extrapyramidal system, and lack of it results in the increased muscle tone of paralysis agitans or Parkinsonism.

Types

(i) Idiopathic

The cause of the degenerative change in the basal ganglia is unknown. This is the common form of this disease, developing insidiously between the ages of 50 and 65, being commoner in men, and there is a slight familial tendency.

(ii) Arteriosclerotic

The degenerative changes are vascular in origin. The condition occurs in the elderly and is accompanied by other evidence of cerebral arteriosclerosis. There may be a history of strokes, and sometimes a degree of dementia.

(iii) Drug-induced

Phenothiazine drugs such as chlorpromazine, and methyldopa, reserpine and metoclopramide, may interfere with the action of dopamine or other neurochemical transmitters. There may be crises of abnormal jerky movements (dystonia) with rigidity and fixed upward gaze of the eyes.

Symptoms and signs

Tremor is often the presenting sign, and is described as a 'pill-rolling' movement or shake of the fingers.

Tremor becomes more marked if the patient is engaged by the examiner in conversation, or is emotionally upset.

It may disappear on performing a voluntary movement and is absent during sleep.

Rigidity of the muscles; the patient has difficulty holding a pen and the writing becomes smaller.

The muscular rigidity causes a 'poverty of movement' with lack of blinking and a loss of the normal facial expression, producing a 'mask-like' face.

A walk with short, shuffling steps.

Voice becomes low and monotonous and all movements are performed slowly.

Though the muscles have increased tone, there are no reflex changes and no true paralysis, rather a restriction of movement.

Bladder function is preserved.

When the forehead of the patient is tapped, he keeps on blinking.

(10) SPINAL CORD COMPRESSION

The spinal cord runs from the foramen magnum of the skull, where it is continuous with the medulla, and ends at the lower level of the first lumbar vertebra. In its course, it gives off and receives the motor and sensory nerve roots, being protected in front by the bodies of the vertebrae (separated by the discs) and surrounded by the neural arches of the vertebrae behind.

Causes of spinal cord damage

(i) Compression
Trauma – following crush fractures, or fracture-dislocation of the vertebrae.

Vertebral disease and spontaneous fracture, as in tumour or myeloma, causing their sudden collapse.

Prolapsed intervertebral disc in the cervical (or dorsal) spine.

Tumour – neurofibroma – may be inside the cord, or affect the meninges or nerve root.

Secondary – metastases from carcinoma (lung, breasts, prostate) or deposits in Hodgkin's disease.

Extradural abscess – often staphylococcal from sepsis elsewhere.

(ii) Arteriosclerosis
Thrombosis of the anterior spinal artery which serves the upper and anterior part of the cord.

(iii) Transverse myelitis
As part of encephalomyelitis.

Symptoms and signs

Transection of the cord above the fourth cervical level is incompatible with life.

Transection at a lower level causes paralysis below the lesion; quadriplegia is paralysis of arms and legs, the more common paraplegia is paralysis of the legs.

Complete loss of sensation below the lesion.

Disturbance of micturition and sometimes defaecation.

Hypotension and loss of sweating.

Further investigations

X-ray of spine (which may show vertebral involvement).

Lumbar puncture: blockage of the CSF circulation may be revealed by compressing each jugular vein in turn, when the normal rise and fall of CSF pressure will be absent. Complete blockage causes yellow CSF with a high protein content, so that it may actually coagulate.

Myelography will localize the level and may indicate the nature of the spinal block.

CAT scan may be helpful in localizing the lesion.

(11) DISORDERS OF THE NERVE ROOTS AND PERIPHERAL NERVES

A nerve fibre can be involved by disease anywhere in its long course from the spinal cord to the periphery. The fault may lie in the nerve cell or its axon (peripheral process), in the insulating myelin sheath, or in the connective tissue binding the fibres to form the nerve trunk. The fault can be the result of many processes: compression and irritation, inflammation, infection and metabolic or vascular upset. Involvement of the nerve fibres leads to impairment of conduction, whether motor or sensory, and this may be followed by degeneration.

The vertebral bodies are separated by the intervertebral discs. With advancing age the discs tend to 'dry', causing stresses on the spinal joints and resulting in a form of degenerative osteoarthritis with the formation of bony outgrowths called 'osteophytes' at the vertebral margins. These encroach on the nerve roots. There is also a varying degree of backward prolapse of the degenerate disc. The process is termed 'spondylosis', and it affects the parts of the spine which have most movement.

(a) CERVICAL SPONDYLOSIS

Symptoms and signs

Irritation and compression of the nerve roots serving the shoulder and arm, usually more marked on one side.

Aching at the neck, and neck movements are restricted.

Muscle spasm and tenderness.

Discomfort, tingling sensation, or pain is felt in the part of the arm served by the affected nerve root or roots, the outer (radial) border of the arm being commonly involved.

There may be some diminution of appreciation of light touch or pin-prick within the affected dermatome (the area of the skin supplied by that nerve), but complete sensory loss is unusual.

There may be some diminution of the tendon reflexes in the arm.

X-rays of the cervical spine will confirm the existence of spondylosis.

(b) ARTHRITIS OF THE LUMBAR SPINE

Symptoms and signs

The degenerative changes in the lumbar spine may be a cause of low backache or lumbago.

May occur acutely after sudden flexion, as in stooping to pick up a heavy weight.

Sudden pain down the back of the thigh and leg – 'sciatica'.

There may be loss of the ankle jerk and pain on attempting to raise the leg to a right angle.

(12) DISORDERS OF PERIPHERAL NERVES

ENTRAPMENT NEUROPATHIES

(a) Cervical

An extra, cervical, rib, or anomalies of structures between the first rib and the clavicle cause narrowing of the cervical outlet, resulting in pressure on the brachial plexus and nerve trunks.

Symptoms and signs

Sensory disturbance usually along the inner (ulnar) border of the arm and hand.

Muscle weakness and wasting.

Symptoms might be worsened by drooping of the shoulder girdle or the carrying of heavy weights.

(b) Carpal tunnel syndrome

The median nerve may be compressed as it passes through the fibrous tunnel at the wrist on its way to serve the hand.

Symptoms and signs

Pain and tingling in the hand and fingers, especially those on the medial side of the hand, often occurring by night.

Discomfort felt at the wrist with tenderness over the fibrous tunnel.

Wasting of the small muscles at the base of the thumb, some of which are supplied by the median nerve.

Common in middle-aged women and is sometimes associated with arthritis or undue use of the wrist.

It may also occur in pregnancy, from fluid retention and tissue swelling; and in myxoedema (hypothyroidism) and acromegaly (a result of hyperpituitarism).

(c) Trauma

In the arm, the radial nerve is very liable to be damaged in its long winding course round the humerus – and it may also be affected in the axilla from prolonged hanging of the arm over a chair ('Saturday night' or 'drunkards' paralysis). The radial nerve is mainly motor, and the lesion results in inability to extend the wrist and fingers.

PERIPHERAL NEUROPATHY

In this group of conditions the peripheral nerves are symmetrically involved. The longer the nerve fibre, the more liable it is to be damaged. Thus there are varying degrees of sensory disturbance and muscular weakness in the feet and limbs.

Causes

(i) Toxic

Lead, arsenic and heavy metals. Lead poisoning (e.g. inhalation of fumes from the burning of car batteries) causes motor-weakness without sensory loss (also constipation, anaemia and a 'blue' lead-line on the gums).

Triorthocresyl phosphate (TOCP) and acrylamide, both used in the plastics industry.

(ii) Deficiency

Vitamin B_1; dry beri-beri may be due to multiple dietary deficiencies rather than deficiency of B_1 alone, and occurs in the

DIFFERENTIAL DIAGNOSIS OF LOSS OF CONSCIOUSNESS

	Onset and duration	*Pre-existing symptoms or conditions*
Intracerebral haemorrhage	abrupt and continuing	hypertension; more common in elderly; headache; hyperthermia later
Subarachnoid haemorrhage	warning headache; abrupt loss of consciousness may be days later	may be minor head injury; headache, neck stiffness; more common in young
Extradural haemorrhage	transient stunning; initial lucid intervals; deepening coma	follows head injury; probable fracture, temporal skull gone; vomiting, drowsiness
Cerebral tumour	slow, preceded by neurological symptoms; loss of consciousness late in disease process	motor, sensory, speech or visual disorder, headache, vomiting or development of convulsions
Syncope	sudden, transient, spontaneous recovery	sweating, psychogenic anxiety, most often in adolescent – young adult
Meningitis	clouding of consciousness slow as disease advances	neck stiffness, fever, vomiting; sepsis focus – e.g. throat, respiratory tract
Epilepsy (grand mal)	abrupt after warning 'aura', tonic and clonic stage, spontaneous recovery; may be frequent, recurrent attacks	more common in young, may be idiopathic or late consequence of skull injury, or cerebral space-occupying lesion

Associated findings	*Key laboratory findings*
hemiplegia; deepening coma, flaccidity of limbs, incontinence of urine; Cheyne–Stokes respiration	blood-stained CSF, increased CSF pressure
flaccid weakness all limbs	CSF heavily blood-stained; brain scan shows site, angiography shows aneurysms
dilated pupil one-sided, flaccid paralysis, papilloedema	brain scan shows space-occupying lesion one side; skull X-ray shows fracture
papilloedema; primary Ca may be in lung; cachexia if metastases	skull X-ray displacement of pineal gland, or fossa erosion; brain scan shows lesion, EEG abnormalities
slow pulse, hypotension, nausea; no neurological abnormalities	all investigations normal
photophobia	lumbar puncture – raised CSF pressure, pus cells, leukocytosis
muscle and limb twitching, violent, incontinence of urine, rigidity of limbs, cyanosis; post-epileptic confusion and amnesia	CSF normal, EEG shows typical 'spike' activity

underdeveloped countries. Alcoholic neuropathy is probably due to similar B vitamin deficiencies, for alcoholics tend to neglect their food, but alcohol may have a direct toxic effect on the nerves. In vitamin B_{12} deficiency peripheral neuropathy can occur.

(iii) Metabolic

Diabetes; loss of sensation at the feet with tendency to ulcer formation, absent vibration sense and reflexes.

Porphyria; a group of conditions due to an inherited disturbance of haemoglobin metabolism or liver defect.

(iv) Infective and inflammatory

Acute infective (ascending) polyneuritis – (Landry–Guillain–Barré syndrome) occurs after infection, especially respiratory infection, or after glandular fever (infections mononucleosis), and may be a disturbance of immunity.

Leprosy.

Diphtheria – due to toxin – paralysis of palate or limbs.

(v) 'Connective-tissue' (collagen-vascular) diseases

'Autoimmune diseases' – group includes rheumatoid arthritis, but polyarteritis nodosa, an inflammation of arteries and nerves affecting middle-aged men, is the usual cause in this group.

(vi) Carcinoma – carcinomatous neuropathy

Carcinoma, especially bronchogenic carcinoma, may be associated with distal sensory changes or sometimes a mixed motor and sensory neuropathy. Cause possibly a toxin produced by the growth.

Symptoms and signs

The sensory disturbance includes complaints such as numbness, paraesthesiae (pins and needles) and pain.

Loss of sensation to pain (pin-prick), temperature and touch.

Often affects feet and ankles, and sometimes the hands, and is described as 'glove and stocking' anaesthesia.

The motor weakness affects the distal muscles causing paralysis of dorsiflexion of the feet and 'foot drop'.

The ankle and knee jerks are absent.

Chapter 9
The Skeletal System

The commonest disorder of the skeletal system will be, with age, osteoarthritis. Musculoskeletal pains cause 10% of all medical consultations, of which one-third will be for backache. Apart from trauma and the effects of ageing, rheumatoid arthritis is the single most frequent disorder of this system that will lead to periodic hospitalization.

Diagnosis of disorder will depend on symptoms, history, observation of the patient and examination of:

(A) X-rays,
(B) blood tests,
(C) biopsy,
(D) arthroscopy.

Common symptoms of generalized disorder will be:

(1) pain,
(2) loss of function, or restricted movement,
(3) swelling of the affected joint(s).

(A) X-RAYS

Straight X-rays of affected joints or bones may reveal abnormalities in porosity, outline or structure. Bone scanning using radioactive isotopes may be necessary to reveal metastases.

(B) BLOOD TESTS

To ascertain white count changes, ESR, uric acid levels and rheumatoid factors are necessary, as are assessment of the blood count, LE latex and antinuclear antibody levels.

(C) BIOPSY

Biopsy of joint or muscle tissue may be necessary to confirm diagnosis, and this can be done at the same time as:

(D) ARTHROSCOPY

The visualization, by means of fibre-optics, of the inside area of affected joints, e.g. the knee.

Common Disorders of the Skeletal System

(1) RHEUMATOID ARTHRITIS

Rheumatoid arthritis is a chronic arthritis of small joints. It may cause only slight disability, or result in crippling deformities. It affects over 3% of the population and is three times commoner in females. It usually presents in young adults in their thirties and forties.

There is inflammation and proliferation of the synovial lining membrane of many joints, which may proceed to cause their destruction.

The fundamental cause is unknown. It is thought that some environmental trigger factor, possibly a virus, stimulates the production of antibodies causing an autoimmune reaction. Immune complexes are deposited in the synovium (and blood vessel walls) causing enzyme release and joint inflammation.

Symptoms and signs

Aching pain.

Stiffness.

Swelling of the joints, especially the smaller joints.

Often worst in the morning, when there is pain and stiffness in the fingers passing off in an hour or two but recurring the next day.

Onset may be acute with severe pain and swelling of joints and tendon sheaths, and the forming of rheumatoid nodules near the elbows.

Constitutional upset includes fever, fatigue, loss of appetite, loss of weight and anaemia.

Further investigations

Rheumatoid factor is detectable in the blood by the Rose Waaler test or the RA (rheumatoid arthritis) latex test.

Blood count shows anaemia, raised white cell count, and high ESR.

X-rays show joint deformity and adjacent bone rarefaction (osteoporosis).

(2) OSTEOARTHRITIS

Osteoarthritis is a degenerative disorder of the larger, weight-bearing joints. It results from a wearing away of the cartilage on the opposite bone surfaces. Trauma and obesity contribute to it, and it is very common in the hips and knees of fat, middle-aged and elderly people. There is no systemic upset, but there may be an associated slight degenerative joint change in the terminal interphalangeal joints of the fingers.

Symptoms and signs

(a) Limb joints

Pain and stiffness with creaking and grating of the large joints, especially after a period of immobility.

Cold and damp may precipitate an attack.

In severe cases there is joint deformity and destruction, and in the hips and knees this can result in serious disability and crippling.

(b) Arthritis of the spine

Changes are especially liable to occur in the cervical spine in association with disc degeneration (cervical spondylosis).

Aches at the neck and restricted movement, often with tenderness and spasm in the surrounding muscles.

Nerve root pressure may cause discomfort in the arms.

Lumbar region arthritis may be associated with the low backache and disc degeneration and prolapse may cause 'sciatica'.

Pain in the distribution of the sciatic nerve at the back of the leg from pressure on the roots contributing to the nerve.

(3) GOUT

A metabolic disease associated with a high blood uric acid, crystals of which are deposited in joints causing recurrent attacks of arthritis.

The high blood uric acid is usually due to an over-production in the body, but there may be a defect in renal tubular excretion in addition. The over-production is a result of abnormal purine metabolism – purines are proteins present in many body cells, especially those of the pancreas and liver. Inherited as a dominant, gout is 95% a male disease, and usually presents after the age of 50. There are racial predispositions, a high uric acid being common in Pacific islanders.

Symptoms and signs

Recurrent attacks of pain and inflammation in one or more joints.

Metatarsophalangeal joint of the big toe is commonly affected.

Symptoms characteristically come on during the night, but may be precipitated by a heavy meal or alcohol, or by an infection or operation.

The pain may be excruciating.

The joint is swollen, red and shiny and exquisitely tender.

Deposits of uric acid may also be seen as white 'tophi' under the skin, especially at the cartilage of the ears.

(4) ANKYLOSING SPONDYLITIS

An inflammatory disease of the joints of the spine, affecting young men. Its cause is unknown but most patients have the HLA group B27.

Symptoms and signs

Occur before the age of 30 and the condition should be suspected in a previously healthy man complaining of backache or pains in the thighs.

The sacroiliac joints are first affected.

Changes are seen on X-ray.

The ESR is raised.

Pain and stiffness of movement of the lumbar spine, spreading up to involve dorsal and even cervical spine.

In later stages bony fixation (ankylosis) of the joints occurs and the patient has a rigid 'poker-back' or 'bamboo spine'.

(5) FIBROSITIS

The term rheumatism is popularly used to mean aches, pains and stiffness attributed to disorders in joints, ligaments or muscles. Inflammatory disease of muscles is not, however, a common cause of recurrent symptoms – the only common inflammation or infection is epidemic myalgia or Bornholm disease, caused by a Coxsackie virus, presenting as chest wall pain and tenderness, and settling within a week or 10 days. Abscesses of muscles may occur in the tropics. Myositis may occur in the rare connective tissue diseases.

When a patient complains of 'rheumatism' or 'fibrositis', it is important to exclude conditions such as the chronic rheumatic disorders, local post-traumatic conditions such as frozen shoulder (inflammation of the tendons and capsule of the shoulder joint), polymyalgia rheumatica and bone disorders. Osteoarthritis of the spine is a common cause of many 'rheumatic' pains. Muscle spasm, from nerve irritation or in an attempt to protect the joint from undue movement, may explain some of the aches and tenderness around the part, and the symptoms are ascribed to the muscles instead of to the causative disease.

The occurrence of symptoms is often ascribed to undue strain, or exposure to draughts, cold and dampness, and a warm climate may improve them. Symptoms are worse in those who are depressed – depressive illness may present with rheumatic pains.

(6) CONNECTIVE TISSUE ('COLLAGEN VASCULAR') DISEASES

A group of diseases in which there is degeneration of connective tissue in association with inflammation of small blood vessels. They may be disturbances of the immune mechanism of the body, and abnormal globulins and antibodies may be detectable in the blood, with a raised ESR.

(a) SYSTEMIC (DISSEMINATED) LUPUS ERYTHEMATOSUS

This relatively rare condition occurs in young women. The cause is unknown but many tissues are involved, possibly from deposition of immune complexes in the small arteries supplying them, with resultant inflammation and degeneration. The condition gets its name from an erythematous rash across the nose and cheeks, a 'butterfly' distribution.

Symptoms and signs

General symptoms include fever and malaise.

Polyarthritis, similar in distribution to rheumatoid arthritis, but more transient.

'Butterfly' erythema at nose and cheeks may be present, often mild but worsened by exposure to sunlight.

Erythema at the nail bases, due to dilated small vessels (telangiectasis), is characteristic.

Purpura may occur.

Thrombosis in small arteries may cause cold, pale fingertips with gangrenous patches.

Acute glomerulonephritis and the risk of renal failure may occur or the more chronic picture of nephrotic syndrome with albuminuria and oedema.

The pleura may be involved, with pleurisy and effusion.

A tendency to haemolytic anaemia.

Increased drug sensitivity with rashes.

Investigations

The white cell count is low, LE latex and antinuclear antibody (ANA) tests in the blood are useful in screening and the DNA binding test (for anti-DNA antibodies) is almost specific. (These tests detect the abnormal antibody in the blood which affects the white cells, some of which engulf others and appear as the typical LE cells on a blood smear.)

ESR is high.

Blood urea may be raised.

(b) POLYARTERITIS NODOSA AND CRANIAL ARTERITIS

Polyarteritis nodosa is a rare disturbance of small arteries throughout the body, commoner in middle-aged men.

Symptoms and signs

Fever.

Tendency to arterial thrombosis with nodulation related to arteries.

Peripheral neuritis.

Raised white cell count with many eosinophilic cells.

High ESR.

May be a patchy recurrent pneumonia.

The diagnosis may be confirmed by muscle biopsy, the blood vessels in the muscle showing characteristic changes.

Structure of bone

Bone contains living cells, in a protein matrix in which calcium salts are deposited. Flat bones such as the sternum, vertebrae and pelvis contain active marrow concerned in blood formation. However, even the long bones are not simply supporting structures, they are metabolically active, calcium deposition and resorption occurring all the time.

Rarefaction of bones occurs in osteoporosis, osteomalacia, hyperparathyroidism, myelomatosis and in metastatic bone disease.

(7) OSTEOPOROSIS

Osteoporosis is a thinning of the bones, a loss of bone density. Normal stresses and strains protect against it, and if a limb is immobilized, osteoporosis occurs. Thus it may be seen locally in the bones round splinted joints, but occurs more generally if a patient is confined to bed. Post-menopausally, it may be due to urinary calcium losses from hormonal deficiency.

Osteoporosis is very common in the elderly. The cause is uncertain. There seems to be a fall in calcium absorption after the age of 70 (possibly due to mild vitamin D deficiency). The hormone calcitonin (secreted mainly in the thyroid and concerned in maintaining the calcium content of the bones) may play a part in osteoporosis.

Symptoms and signs

Osteoporosis especially affects the spine, the vertebrae becoming smaller, so that elderly people do become shorter in stature and may have prominent transverse skin-creases across the abdomen.

There are aches and pains in the back.

Fracture of the neck of the femur, a common result of a fall in the elderly, may be more liable to occur if there is osteoporosis.

(8) METASTATIC BONE DISEASE

Malignant secondary deposits (metastases) are a common cause of bone disease. Bone aches and pains occur – symptoms may precede those of the primary tumour. X-ray changes are late, but bone scanning using radioactive isotopes may allow earlier detection. Spontaneous 'pathological' fractures may occur, and in the spine these may cause cord compression and paraplegia.

The primary site may be in the prostate, breast, thyroid or lung.

(9) DISEASES OF MUSCLE – MYOPATHY

(a) THE MUSCULAR DYSTROPHY GROUP (INHERITED MYOPATHIES)

This is a group of rare, hereditary disorders affecting mainly young people, and causing muscular weakness.

Types

Duchenne type – pseudohypertrophic muscular dystrophy. Presents in infancy, occurs only in boys – it is a sex-linked recessive disorder. Waddling gait, weakness and tendency to contractures, muscles appear bulky but become progressively paralysed – child rises from the floor by 'climbing stairs' – and progressively weaker over 10–20 years.

Limb-girdle type – adolescents affected, both sexes, autosomal recessive, weakness of shoulder and in raising arms, difficulty climbing stairs – progressively weaker over 10–20 years.

Facio-scapulo-humeral type – less severe and may present in adults – autosomal dominant inheritance so that affected individuals pass it on to half their children. Weakness of facial muscles and difficulty in closing the eyes and puffing the

DIFFERENTIAL DIAGNOSIS OF JOINT PAINS

	Site, onset and duration	*Pre-existing symptoms or conditions*
Rheumatoid arthritis	small joints affected, gradual and continual deterioration, permanent, crippling	commoner in females, predominantly develops in 30–40-year-olds; bouts of fever, fatigue, anorexia
Osteoarthritis	larger weight-bearing joints, continual restriction of mobility	overweight and elderly; no systemic upset
Gout	usually an isolated joint affected – big toe commonest; worse at night; recurrent attacks with remissions	predominantly male adults, may be precipitated by alcohol
Septic arthritis	any joint, follows systemic disease or injury; resolution depending on extent of local destruction	pyogenic, tuberculous or gonococcal infection precedes; fever, anorexia, malaise
Traumatic arthritis	any joint, recovery depends on extent of injury	history of trauma, rapid development with 24 h of symptoms; no systemic upset

Associated findings	*Key laboratory findings*
morning stiffness, rheumatic nodules, joint deformity and inflammation	anaemia, Rh factor present, high ESR, WBC raised, X-ray shows joint deformity and osteoporosis
continual joint movement restriction; swelling of joint, non-inflammatory	X-rays show bone deformity, osteophytes, destruction of articular surface; ESR normal
'tophic' deposits in ear cartilage; swollen red joint extremely painful to touch or movement	raised serum uric acid, abnormal purine metabolism results, uric acid crystals in joint aspirate
all movement painful, single red swollen joint	cytology and culture of aspirate confirms causative organism; ESR, WBC raised; may be proteinuria
swollen joint, loss of movement, pain increases after initial injury	blood tests normal, X-ray may show fracture or, under stress, ligament tear

cheeks, winging of scapulae, some weakness in arms and legs with tendency to waddling gait. Often remains in this mild form over many years.

Investigations

Serum enzymes – creatine kinase raised in Duchenne type.

Electromyography – investigation of electrical activity of the muscles, which is disturbed.

Muscle biopsy.

(b) ENDOCRINE, METABOLIC AND CARCINOMATOUS MYOPATHIES

Proximal myopathy, weakness of the muscles of the shoulder-girdle and thigh, may complicate thyroid disorders (thyrotoxicosis, myxoedema). The patient has difficulty in raising the arms above the head, and in stair climbing. There may be wasting of the affected muscles.

A low serum potassium level (hypokalaemia) causes muscular weakness, and occurs in aldosteronism, but the excessive use of diuretics is the commonest reason.

Rare defects of muscle sugars and enzyme abnormalities are associated with muscle weakness.

Carcinoma, especially bronchogenic carcinoma, may be associated with myasthenia-like muscle weakness and should be considered in the middle-aged and elderly.

(10) MYASTHENIA GRAVIS

An uncommon disease with onset in adult life or late childhood. There is a defect in the transmission of the nerve impulse at the neuromuscular junction so that the muscle fails to contract and remains flaccid.

The disease is due to destruction of the acetylcholine receptors at the neuromuscular junction and antibodies to this receptor are demonstrable in the blood – thus it is an autoimmune disease. The disturbance of immunity may be related to a defective thymus gland, which may be enlarged or, in some cases, contain a tumour.

Symptoms and signs

The patient experiences muscle weakness, especially of muscles of the face, so that he may have difficulty in keeping his eyes open, in chewing, and even in swallowing.

The arms may also be affected.

Symptoms are worse towards the end of the day when the muscles are tired.

Diagnosis and treatment

The diagnosis is confirmed by the slow intravenous injection of edrophonium 10 mg, a cholinergic drug which produces an immediate return of muscular power.

Plasmaphoresis, a technique of filtering the blood plasma to remove the acetylcholine receptor antibody, is diagnostic.

Chapter 10
The Skin

Disorders of the skin are common, a frequent cause of consultation but an infrequent cause of hospitalization and an exceptionally rare cause of death. Acute and chronic infections, eczema, dermatitis, allergic rashes and the rare skin tumour are the main disorders and more than 15% of the population, in all age groups, will seek medical attention in each year.

Diagnosis of disorder will depend on symptoms, signs, observation of the patient (particularly) and examination of:
(A) the skin,
(B) blood tests,
(C) urine tests,
(D) biopsy.

Common symptoms of generalized disorder will be:
(1) a localized, or generalized, rash,
(2) swelling,
(3) pain,
(4) itching.

Common Disorders of the Skin

(1) INFECTIONS

(a) BACTERIAL

Boils are due to staphylococcal infection in a hair follicle and may go on to abscess or carbuncle formation.

Impetigo is an infection caused by staphylococci and streptococci together, and consists of blisters, tending to become pustular and crusted, on inflamed skin. It may follow neglect, scratching and lack of cleanliness after abrasions or septic spots, and is seen mainly in children.

Erysipelas is a spreading inflammation in the superficial layers of the skin near a mucocutaneous junction such as the lips or nose. It is a streptococcal infection.

Cellulitis is a spreading inflammation in the subcutaneous tissues from a septic area or ulcer. The cause is usually a staphylococcal or streptococcal infection.

(b) FUNGUS

Infection of the mouth with the fungus *Candida (Monilia)* results in the white patches called thrush, which is found in debilitated patients or those receiving broad-spectrum antibiotics. A similar infection may occur in the vagina, causing pruritus vulvae, and is especially likely to occur in diabetics and women using oral contraceptives.

Intertrigo is a moist red rash occurring where two surfaces rub together and cleanliness is lacking, and may be due to an eczema reaction complicated by a low-grade infection with a fungus of the *Candida* group. It is common under the breasts of obese women – there is an offensive oozing patch with a red edge containing pinpoint vesicles.

Tinea is a term applied to other human fungus infections of the skin; conditions sometimes called ringworm. In children, ringworm may affect the hair; but in adults the condition is seen in moist areas – between the toes (athlete's foot) and at the groins. Between the toes the skin becomes soggy and macerated. At the groins there is a spreading red ring (which gives the disease its name) of inflammation, with healing tending to occur in the centre of the patch – the same appearance as intertrigo, with considerable irritation and some odour. Tinea can also affect the nails. Other forms of ringworm are acquired from contact with infected animals.

(c) VIRUS

Herpes simplex is a virus infection, causing 'cold sores' around the lips and nose, sometimes in association with lobar pneumonia. It may also attack the genital area.

Herpes zoster (shingles) is a vesicular eruption along the line of a nerve – seen usually on the trunk, sometimes in the face from involvement of the ophthalmic division of the fifth cranial (trigeminal) nerve. Pain may be severe, with tendency to secondary infection. The virus responsible also causes chickenpox, yet contact spread is rare.

Molluscum contagiosum is a virus infection causing little water blisters; it may be acquired at swimming pools.

Common warts are induced by virus infection, though the reasons for their appearances and disappearances are obscure.

(2) INFESTATIONS

(a) LOUSE INFESTATION (PEDICULOSIS)

Lice are small flat insects which feed on blood. Head lice may infest the scalp of children, young women and youths with long hair, the eggs or nits being attached to the shaft of the hair. The nits are greyish-white specks and in severe infestation the hair may be covered with them. The irritation of the adult lice causes scratching and minor skin infection, with enlargement of the occipital and cervical lymph glands as a result. Infestation spreads easily in schools.

Body lice affect people who are dirty – vagrants, and those living in squalid conditions. The bites appear as small red spots, and there is much scratching and slight secondary infection. The louse lives in the seams of clothing, where it lays its eggs.

Crab lice affect the pubic region and are spread by sexual intercourse.

(b) SCABIES

Scabies is an infestation with a small mite called the acarus. The female acarus is just visible to the naked eye and burrows into the epidermis, causing severe itching. Favourite sites are the clefts of the fingers, the front of the wrists and elbows, axillary fold and pectoral region – areas which can be scratched, the parasite being spread by the fingernails. The burrows are visible as greyish lines up to a centimetre in length and there may be a raised red eruption which tends to secondary infection. Minor epidemics of scabies occur in schoolchildren and in the elderly in hospital, the condition being very contagious in institutions. The acarus can be picked out with a pin and identified under the microscope.

(c) FLEAS

Flea bites cause itchy raised red spots with a central bite-mark.

(3) DERMATITIS AND ECZEMA

Dermatitis means inflammation of the skin and includes the 'eczema reaction' which typically starts with erythema (reddening) followed by the formation of tiny fluid-containing vesicles and 'weeping' followed by a more chronic scaling stage when the skin may become thickened or 'lichenified'. Eczematous lesions are usually extremely itchy. The terms dermatitis and eczema are sometimes used interchangeably.

Eczema may be present in infancy and be followed by flexural eczema in childhood. There is an association with asthma, and such patients are said to manifest atopy, an inherited tendency to show hypersensitivity or allergic reactions. The eczema and asthma may improve in adolescence, but the skin seems to remain very sensitive. People with no previous allergic history may also have skins which are prone to show the eczema reaction. Chemicals and drugs cause contact dermatitis in susceptible subjects. Soaps and detergents, and substances met with at work (occupational or industrial dermatitis) may cause contact dermatitis.

Some patients are prone to a form of eczema, called seborrhoeic eczema or seborrhoeic dermatitis, occurring especially in flexures, e.g. behind the ears causing fissuring, in the axillae, groins or under the breasts. Seborrhoea means increased sebum and there is an association with dandruff and dermatitis near the hair follicles.

(4) DRUG RASHES

These are very common and while the eruption may follow local application or contact, usually it is due to a drug that has been taken by mouth. Drug eruptions are a result of a delayed hypersensitivity, a cell-mediated allergic reaction.

Barbiturates, especially phenobarbitone, may provoke a diffuse blotchy-red itchy rash, or many red spots tending to coalesce rather like measles.

Aspirin, sulphonamides, antibiotics especially ampicillin, and oral anticoagulants such as phenindione may cause a skin eruption in sensitive subjects.

Iodine-containing substances, used in X-ray contrast media and in proprietary cough treatment, may cause a characteristic vesicular rash.

Heavy metals such as gold, used in the treatment of rheumatoid arthritis, may cause a severe exfoliative dermatitis (erythroderma) with generalized reddening of the skin, and there may be extensive peeling.

(5) URTICARIA

This is the appearance of itchy red lumps in the skin, from oedema and inflammation in the deeper layer (dermis). In some cases the patient, using his fingernails or a match-stick, may be able to write his name on his skin.

Some individuals have this heightened reactivity when exposed to nervous stress, such as examinations, to a hot or cold bath or to contact with or ingestion of substances ranging

DIFFERENTIAL DIAGNOSIS OF SKIN RASHES

	Site, onset and duration	*Pre-existing symptoms or conditions*
Bacteriological infections	local, rapid development, often follicular or following injury; may be boil or confluent sepsis	debilitation or self-neglect, acne, evidence of contagion, recurrent attacks
Fungus infections	oral, vaginal or intertrigo, slow development, recurrent and resistant to therapy	may be using oral contraceptive, antibiotics (broad-spectrum) or diabetic; animal contact with some tineas, or family spread
Virus infections	may be single papilloma – wart – or widespread viraemia typical of measles, rubella, chickenpox; herpes-specific rash on lips, as zoster following nerve root, or on genitalia	if viraemia, often previous signs of URTI and coryza, fever, headache, anorexia, photophobia; 'Koplik's' oral spots of measles
Eczema	flexures of limbs initially, may spread; may occur where skin in contact with 'sensitizer'; worse in atopy, seasonally	atopics have history of asthma, contact dermatitis response caused by occupational exposure; seborrhoea; strong family history
Urticaria	may be widespread, only perioral, or on 'exposed' skin areas; onset rapid, progress to wheal and 'target', spontaneous resolution	allergic history, may be initiated by known allergen, e.g. salicylates, foodstuff, etc., or cold exposure; psychogenic response; affects the young and female mostly
Psoriasis	scalp, elbows and knees – may be discrete or confluent areas elsewhere on body	often presents in adolescent, genetic recessive, therefore strong family history

Associated findings	*Key laboratory findings*
pustular, crusted discharge, lymphadenopathy; painful erythema surrounds	raised WBC, culture of discharge confirms organism; check for glycosuria
itches and then becomes painful to stretching; may bleed; ringworm typical in appearance; tinea may be moist with skin flake shedding; nail changes in some	normal blood tests check for glycosuria; mycelium grown on culture or seen in skin scrapings under microscopy
lymphadenopathy herpes accompanies skin temperature elevation. No itching until crusted rash of chicken-pox or herpes develops	ESR raised, WBC and specific anti-body changes; cytology of chickenpox lesions unnecessary if diagnostic rash distribution
itching, exudative, crusting rash; 'typical' distribution, allergic family or personal history of migraine, urticaria, hay fever, etc.	eosinophilia, immunoglobulin changes
itching, may be severe, with localized oedema; sometimes temporarily arthritic findings	occasional immunoglobulin changes; may show evidence of parasitic infestation (intestinal)
fingernail pitting, sometimes destructive small joint arthropathy; non-itchy, scaly rash; improves with UVL	typical microscopic pattern of biopsied lesion; X-ray shows bilateral arthropathies

from tomatoes to drugs, or following insect bites.

Severe cases go on to 'angioneurotic oedema' when there is a puffy oedematous swelling of the eyes and face, and the larynx may also become swollen from oedema.

(6) PSORIASIS

A common chronic skin disease, often presenting in adolescence, but it may occur at any age. It is characterized by scaly patches on the skin. The cause is unknown but there is a familial tendency, and although the lesions appear discrete, there is a disturbance of function throughout the epidermis.

The scaly patches often occur over extensor surfaces such as elbows and knees but in severe cases may be much more diffuse. The patches are disc-sized or larger, reddish and slightly raised, the scales producing a silvery appearance with a white line on scraping. The condition is unsightly, with much flaking of the scales, but there need be no itch. Psoriasis may be associated with an arthritis rather like rheumatoid arthritis, though the terminal joints of the fingers are more liable to be involved and psoriasis of the nails may be associated.

(7) TUMOURS OF THE SKIN

(a) PRIMARY TUMOURS

The rodent ulcer or basal cell carcinoma is a slow-growing tumour occurring on the face near the nose, eye or ear of an elderly person.

A squamous cell carcinoma is a more rapidly growing malignancy which spreads to lymph nodes.

The common mole or naevus rarely becomes malignant, but the malignant melanoma is a pigmented spot of high malignancy which spread locally, and metastasizes commonly to the liver.

(b) SECONDARY TUMOURS

Secondary deposits present as little lumps in the skin, which may ulcerate. The primary is commonly a carcinoma of the lung or stomach. Skin involvement means that the spread is extensive and the outlook poor, with only palliative treatment being possible.

Skin deposits may also occur in leukaemia and the reticuloses.

Acanthosis nigricans is a dark scaly eruption which is a reaction to carcinoma. The tumour may not be clinically manifest, but the appearance of the characteristic skin eruption should lead to a search for its presence.

Chapter 11
The Endocrine–Hormonal System

The commonest disorder of the endocrine–hormonal metabolic system is diabetes, with thyroid, adrenal and pituitary disorders following in order of frequency. They account for at least 2% of all hospital admissions and all increase in incidence with age.

Diagnosis of disorder will depend on symptoms, history, observation of the patient and examination of:
(A) blood tests,
(B) urine tests.

Common symptoms of generalized disorder will be:
(1) loss (or gain) of weight,
(2) frequency of urination,
(3) fatigue (or excitability),
(4) anorexia.

(A) BLOOD TESTS

These will be complicated, depending on the disorder being investigated. Hormonal level estimation in blood has only comparatively recently been made available through procedures such as electrophoresis, chromatography and radioisotope tests – although blood sugar estimation has been practicable for many years.

(B) URINE TESTS

Assessment for glycosuria has been made for centuries – the development of enzyme strip tests and special tablet tests has revolutionized the more accurate measurement. Hormonal output analysis is, nevertheless, much more complicated and primarily an achievement of the comprehensively equipped laboratory.

Common Disorders of the Endocrine–Hormonal System

(1) DIABETES

Diabetes mellitus is a disorder of metabolism characterized by a high blood sugar and the passage of large quantities of sugar-containing urine.

Cause of diabetes mellitus

Diabetes is due to a relative or absolute deficiency of insulin action. Insulin is the pancreatic hormone.

The pancreas has two component parts – the exocrine digestive enzyme-secreting part, and the endocrine part, the islets of Langerhans. Insulin is secreted into the bloodstream by the cells of the islets. The stimulus to insulin secretion is a high blood sugar level acting directly on the pancreas, but glucose and amino acids in the upper intestine after a meal also stimulate insulin secretion indirectly by the action of certain gut hormones on the pancreas.

In diabetes, the secretion of insulin is deranged. In the severe diabetes of the young the cells are very defective and there is a lack of insulin production. In older diabetics, who are frequently obese, the plasma insulin may be higher than in a thin, normal person, but there is a deficiency of secretion relative to needs.

Diabetes sometimes runs in families, but the genetic basis is not clear and is probably multifactorial. There is some evidence of an association with Coxsackie virus infection, but there is as yet no proof of a virus cause in most cases.

Insulin antagonists, pituitary- or adrenal-dependent, have been thought to be operative. The muscles of the obese may have a metabolic block in glucose uptake (which is sidetracked to the fat depots) which increases insulin demands. Blood vessel abnormalities occur in diabetes, and altered permeability of capillaries might impair insulin passage. All these factors create an increased demand on the pancreas to produce insulin, and while this demand may be met for many years, ultimately it results in pancreatic exhaustion and clinical diabetes.

Insulin is necessary for glucose and amino acids to cross cell membranes; where it is deficient, the body cells cannot properly utilize carbohydrates, fats and proteins. The upset in carbohydrate metabolism is the obvious manifestation, with high blood glucose and glycosuria, but it is only one aspect of a profound metabolic disturbance.

Incidence

The highest recorded population incidence is 40% in the Pima Indians in Arizona aged 45 or older, and there is a high incidence of a type of diabetes in West Africa. Generally, there is an association of diabetes with high calorie intake and obesity. Clinical diabetes exists in about 2% of the population of the UK and USA.

Diabetes is rare in infancy, quite common in childhood and adolescence in both sexes, but most commonly presents in patients beyond middle-age, especially women.

Clinical types

Type 1

Juvenile, growth-onset, ketotic, 'insulin-dependent' group.

The onset is in childhood or young adult life, symptoms are severe and often acute, the patients are thin, lose weight and are prone to ketoacidosis (excess production of ketone bodies such as acetone and acids from fat breakdown) and coma.

Type 2

Maturity-onset, adult, non-ketotic, 'non-insulin-dependent' group. These are middle-aged or elderly people, commonly women, who are or have been obese. The clinical symptoms may be mild, the condition often presenting as a diabetic 'complication' such as a septic foot sore, and ketosis is unusual.

At some time the unduly large food intake of these patients caused pancreatic stimulation and plenty of insulin was produced, but ultimately the pancreas cannot quite keep up with the demand, and symptoms result. In a proportion of patients the pancreas may remain unable to produce quite enough insulin, but responds to stimulation with an oral sulphonylurea drug such as chlorpropamide.

Symptoms and signs

The diabetic patient cannot utilize glucose. It therefore builds up in the bloodstream (hyperglycaemia), and is excreted in the urine.

Polyuria.

The excessive water loss causes severe thirst, and dehydration if the patient does not slake his thirst.

There is loss of weight despite a good appetite, and muscular weakness.

In the severe diabetes of the young, the body breaks down fats instead of sugar in an attempt to maintain energy processes. These breakdown products are the 'ketone bodies' acetone and keto-acids, which build up in the blood (and spill into the urine) and are toxic to the brain. Ketosis or keto-acidosis is one form of acidosis.

The patient becomes drowsy and ill, with vomiting,

dehydration, and air-hunger; his breath also smelling of acetone.

Diabetic coma may occur.

Complications

Vascular disease

Diabetics are prone to develop arteriosclerosis (atherosclerosis), the degenerative disease of the lining of the arteries, related probably to the disturbed lipid (fat) metabolism. There is a raised incidence of coronary and cerebral arterial disease, and involvement of the leg arteries is very common – including symptoms such as intermittent claudication – but the distal arteries may be more affected, leading to gangrene of the toes and feet.

Eye disease

Retinopathy is the most serious ocular complication of diabetes, and the single most common cause of blindness among the middle-aged. Some years after the diagnosis of diabetes, little aneurysms and haemorrhages related to the retinal capillaries and veins become visible with the ophthalmoscope, and sometimes 'exudates' are seen. These may involve an important part of the retina, causing visual impairment.

Renal disease

There are capillary changes in the renal glomeruli where they become abnormally permeable resulting in proteinuria, usually slight, but occasionally severe, with nephrotic syndrome and oedema, progressing to renal destruction and uraemia.

Neuropathy

Peripheral neuritis or neuropathy may occur in poorly controlled diabetes, with pains and paraesthesiae (pins and needles) and sensory loss; the patient may burn or injure his feet without being aware of it. There is loss of vibration sensation, loss of ankle and knee jerks; there may be muscular weakness.

Infections

Pruritus and vulval irritation are due to infection with the fungus *Candida (Monilia) albicans*, thrush, which may feed on the sugar deposited from the urine.

Skin sepsis and carbuncles, often staphylococcal, are common.

THE DIAGNOSIS OF DIABETES — URINE AND BLOOD TESTS

Glucose

(a) *Qualitative tests.* Clinistix, Tes-tape, and compound strips such as Multistix – the test area on these strips is specific for glucose.
(b) *Quantitative tests.* Clinitest tablets are based on the same principle. Having established the presence of glucose with a preliminary strip test, the Clinitest test allows an estimation of its quantity, thus:

orange-red, 2%	– urine full of sugar
yellow-brown, 1%	– considerable sugar
green, ½%	– slight sugar
blue, nil	– no sugar.

In the management of diabetes, it is important to test specimens freshly produced by the kidneys and corresponding to the blood at the time; thus a true 'morning urine' is obtained by voiding the bladder on wakening and discarding this urine (which has lain in the bladder all night), then passing a fresh specimen ½–1 h later for test.

Ketones are detected by the Acetest tablet or Ketostix strip.

In severe diabetes the urine, though pale, is of high specific gravity from its glucose content.

Blood tests

The terms blood sugar and blood glucose are synonymous.

In health the fasting blood glucose is less than 5.5 mmol/l (100 mg/dl) and even after food seldom rises about 6.7 mmol/l (120 mg/dl). In most people glucose does not appear in the urine until the blood glucose is over 10.0 mmol/l (180 mg/dl), the renal threshold for glucose. Some normal people have a low renal threshold and a 'renal leak' for glucose – renal glycosuria. In the elderly, the renal threshold may be raised.

In the presence of other clinical signs, a casual blood glucose level of over 10 mmol/l (180 mg/dl) confirms the diagnosis of diabetes without need for further tests.

In doubtful cases a glucose tolerance test is carried out. The patient takes his meals normally the day before, but has nothing to eat on the morning of the tests. A fasting blood glucose specimen is taken then 75 g of glucose or the equivalent quantity of liquid glucose is drunk in 5 min in 200–500 ml of flavoured water. Further specimens for glucose estimation are taken after ½ h, 1 h and 2 h. In diabetes the fasting blood glucose level is usually raised and the subsequent levels which can be plotted as a graph or 'curve', rise very high, sometimes up to 20 mmol/l (360 mg/dl), and fail to return to the fasting level in 2 h as in the normal. The diagnosis of diabetes is made if the fasting blood glucose concentration is 7 mmol/l (126 mg/dl) or over, or the 2 h level is 10 mmol/l (180 mg/dl) or over.

The Dextrostix strip test is a most useful screening test of the blood glucose level: a drop of blood is placed on the test area, washed off after a minute, and the grey colour compared with

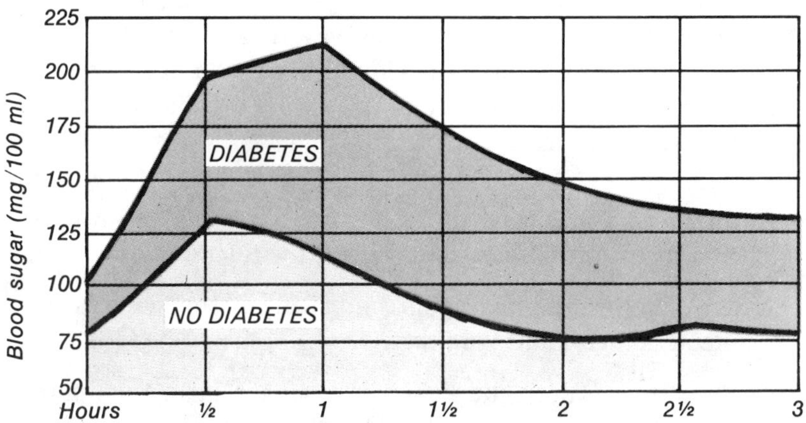

Glucose tolerance curves of diabetic and non-diabetic

a set of standards. The range for visual estimation is 0–14 mmol/l (250 mg/dl). It is difficult to be accurate at the higher levels with the naked eye, but portable instruments such as a reflectance meter are available.

ACUTE COMPLICATIONS OF DIABETES

(i) Hypoglycaemia

This is really a complication of therapy, too much insulin causing an excessive drop in the blood glucose level.

Symptoms and signs

The onset may follow unaccustomed exertion or activity, or a missed meal.

There is sudden weakness, unsteadiness, dizzy feelings, with tremulousness and sweating from outpouring of adrenaline as the body attempts to raise the blood glucose by breaking down liver glycogen.

The patient may become disorientated and violent before collapsing in coma.

(ii) Diabetic ketoacidosis (ketosis) and coma

Diabetic ketosis is a condition of gradual onset, though a young diabetic may present in this way. In a known diabetic, ketosis follows a period of inadequate insulin dosage, and this may have followed infection or stress, which create an increased insulin requirement.

Symptoms and signs

The patient is dehydrated and thirsty, the tongue is dry.

Often there is abdominal pain simulating appendicitis or an 'acute abdomen', and vomiting.

The breathing is deep and sighing (air hunger) in an attempt to excrete the acids as carbon dioxide from the lungs.

The blood pressure falls.

The level of consciousness deteriorates with coma.

There will have been a stage of polyuria, though oliguria may have followed.

The urine is full of glucose and ketones.

(2) THYROID DISORDERS

The thyroid gland consists of a left and right lobe lying against the lower half of the thyroid cartilage, united by a isthmus across the front of the trachea. It secretes the iodine-containing hormone, thyroxine, a metabolic stimulant acting on many tissues.

(a) SIMPLE GOITRE

This may be due to iodine deficiency in endemic areas; the addition of tiny quantities of iodine to salt is preventive. However, simple goitre is not always due to iodine deficiency and may have a genetic basis. Slight thyroid enlargement is common in pregnancy, related to increased iodine demands.

Simple goitre is a soft swelling of the thyroid gland and is commonest in young women. It may be regarded as an attempt by the thyroid to produce enough of its hormone secretion by enlarging.

(b) THYROTOXICOSIS – HYPERTHYROIDISM ('GRAVES' DISEASE') – TOXIC GOITRE

This is overactivity of the thyroid gland, the excess thyroxine causing increased metabolism. Thyrotoxicosis may be a disturbance of the immune mechanism, an autoimmune disease.

Thyrotoxicosis is commoner in women and there is a familial tendency.

Symptoms and signs

The patient complains of excitability, 'nerves' and irritability and may notice that she loses her temper more easily than before.

She feels the heat badly and prefers cold weather.

The palms are warm and sweaty and there is a tremor of the fingers.

The pulse is rapid.

The appetite remains good, the patient may say that she 'eats like a horse', but there is loss of weight from the increased metabolism.

With the stethoscope a 'bruit' may be audible over an enlarged thyroid, from the increased blood flow.

There is a varying degree of 'exophthalmos'. Exophthalmos is protrusion of the eyeball, but the term is used to describe prominence of the eyes. The commonest sign is a 'staring' appearance from overactivity of the sympathetic nervous system which supplies a small muscle in the upper lid, causing lid retraction. There is 'lid lag' on eye movement so that more of the white sclera is seen and the eyes appear prominent.

Investigations

The diagnosis is confirmed by:

(1) Clinical features such as weight loss and raised sleeping pulse.
(2) Raised T_4, corresponding to thyroxine, and estimated by radioimmunoassay in the blood.
(3) TRH test – an injection of TRH normally releases TSH (thyroid stimulating hormone) from the pituitary but in thyrotoxicosis the TSH is already suppressed by the high thyroid activity and the blood level does not rise.
(4) High uptake of radioactive iodine (^{131}I or ^{125}I) over the thyroid gland.

(c) MYXOEDEMA – HYPOTHYROIDISM – UNDERACTIVITY OF THE THYROID GLAND

In the newborn baby the thyroid gland may function defectively or be absent. Early diagnosis is essential and screening tests at birth for blood thyroxine or TSH levels are necessary.

In adults hypothyroidism usually follows destruction of the thyroid gland by an autoimmune process, and antibodies are detectable in the blood. At some stage there may have been swelling and lymphocyte infiltration of the thyroid – (Hashimoto's disease); the condition ends up as atrophy, with complete lack of thyroxine, and the clinical picture called myxoedema.

Symptoms and signs

The condition is commonest in middle-aged women.

As the thyroid fails to produce enough thyroxine, the bodily functions generally run down.

The patient loses interest in life and becomes slower with coarsening and puffiness of the facial appearance and skin.

Characteristically slow relaxation of the tendon reflexes.

Patients become increasingly sluggish, have a husky voice and feel the cold badly.

The pulse is slow, and there may be pericardial effusion.

Investigations

The diagnosis is confirmed by a low blood thyroid index and a raised TSH (thyroid stimulating hormone, from compensatory pituitary activity). Thyroid antibodies may be detected. The serum cholesterol is high.

(3) PARATHYROID DISORDERS

These four glands, situated behind the thyroid, control calcium and phosphorus metabolism, preserving the normal blood calcium level. Excess parathyroid hormone raises the blood calcium by action on kidneys and bones.

(A) HYPOPARATHYROIDISM

This may occur spontaneously or following inadvertent removal of the parathyroids at thyroid operation.

Symptoms and signs

The blood calcium falls, causing increased irritability of nerves with painful muscle cramps and spasm-tetany.

There is painful flexion of the wrists with metacarpophalangeal joints, with extension of the fingers.

There may also be spasm of the larynx.

Tapping over the facial nerve produces twitching of the facial muscles.

Tetany may be provoked by over-breathing, leading to loss of carbon dioxide and tendency to alkalosis.

(B) HYPERPARATHYROIDISM

Overactivity is usually due to a benign tumour of one parathyroid gland. It is rarely palpable. Radioisotope scan (using labelled methionine) may aid in its location.

Symptoms and signs

In severe cases, calcium is dissolved from the bones, producing osteitis fibrosa cystica, and fractures.

Calcium is high in the blood and urine, and may be deposited in the kidneys and cause renal calculi.

There is often polyuria.

Raised serum calcium.

(4) ADRENAL GLAND DISORDERS

The adrenal or suprarenal glands are situated one on top of each kidney. The adrenal gland has a cortex, essential to life, and a medulla which functions independently producing adrenaline-like hormones. The cortex produces three groups of hormones:

(1) Hydrocortisone (cortisol) – a glucocorticoid – so called because it increases protein breakdown resulting in increased production of glucose; essential for normal

response to stress and injury; also has sodium-retaining action.

(2) Aldosterone, concerned in sodium and water balance through its action on the renal tubule. Causes sodium retention.

(3) Sex hormones, which are dominantly masculinizing (androgenic) even in women.

(a) OVERACTION

(i) Overproduction of cortisol

This is usually due to pituitary overactivity, with excessive production of ACTH which causes bilateral adrenal enlargement and overproduction of cortisol.

Symptoms and signs

There is 'mooning' of the face which is often high-coloured.

Obesity of the trunk with thinning of arms and legs.

Muscular weakness.

Thinning of the skin with easy bruising.

Thinning of the bones causing osteoporosis and sometimes fractures.

Hypertension and diabetes mellitus.

Investigations

The diagnosis is confirmed by raised urinary and blood cortisol levels throughout the 24 h (blood levels are normally lower late at night), and raised ACTH (estimated by radioimmunoassay) if there is primary pituitary overactivity.

(ii) Aldosteronism

Primary aldosteronism is due to a tumour, usually benign, producing excess aldosterone, causing hypertension, weakness and polyuria. The serum potassium is low, and the blood shows a tendency to alkalosis.

Secondary aldosteronism occurs when there is a threat of a

lowered plasma volume, as in nephrotic syndrome and cirrhosis of the liver; it may also occur in congestive cardiac failure. It results in salt and water retention with increased oedema.

(iii) Adrenal virilism

This is due to inappropriate production of masculinizing sex hormone by the adrenal cortex. It may cause precocious puberty, or difficulties in sexual designation of infants who are really female but appear male. Cases in adults arc usually due to malignant tumours of the adrenal.

The urine contains an excess of hormone breakdown products, measured as 17-ketosteroids (oxosteroids).

(b) UNDERACTION

Addison's disease

This is a result of deficiency of cortisol and aldosterone.

Symptoms and signs

Loss of appetite and of weight.

Vomiting.

Low blood pressure.

There is a brown pigmentation of the skin, well seen in flexures (e.g. axilla) and scars and in the forehead at the hair line. (The cortisol deficiency causes an increased secretion of ACTH by the pituitary and this is associated with increased secretion of MSH, a hormone which stimulates the production of the melanin pigment.)

There is progressive weakness, with poor resistance to stress and infection.

Investigations

The serum sodium may be low and the potassium and blood urea raised.

Plasma cortisol assessment is necessary.

Patients with underactivity of the adrenal cortex have a low plasma cortisol level and in cases due to primary adrenal disease, i.e. Addison's disease, it fails to rise after ACTH. The blood is taken for test before, and ½ h after, injection.

Side-effects of cortisone-like (corticosteroid or steroid) drugs

Cortisol (hydrocortisone) is essential to life, and the adrenal cortex secretes about 30–40 mg daily. More is required to cover the stress of injury or infection. Apart from its replacement role, cortisol (or cortisone, which is changed to cortisol in the body) can be used pharmacologically in much bigger dosage to treat conditions such as severe asthma and status asthmaticus, overwhelming septicaemias, haemolytic anaemia, and disturbances of immunity. But inseparable from such beneficial action are undesirable actions which would ultimately result in a 'moon' face, muscle weakness, thinning of the bones, hypertension, tendency to diabetes and possible worsening of peptic ulceration.

In an attempt to avoid such effects, synthetic steroids similar to cortisol have been produced. These include prednisone and prednisolone, 5 mg equalling 25 mg cortisone in potency. These drugs may have less of the salt-retaining, hypertensive properties of cortisone, but usage effects will still be seen in long-continued dosage.

Moreover, such steroids will inhibit production of pituitary ACTH, so that the body's own adrenal cortex becomes atrophic, and if the administered steroid is then withdrawn, the patient will pass into a state of adrenal cortical insufficiency with hypotension and collapse.

(c) THE ADRENAL MEDULLA

Phaeochromocytoma is a tumour which secretes excess adrenaline or noradrenaline – the hormones released at sympathetic nerve endings.

There is hypertension, often paroxysmal, severe sweating and pallor.

The tumour may be palpable, or detectable at IVP or on X-ray after retroperitoneal injection of gas.

Adrenaline breakdown products (catecholamines) are detected in a 24 h urine collection.

(5) PITUITARY GLAND DISORDERS

The pituitary is a small gland (about the size of a pea), situated in a fossa at the base of the skull. Above it is the optic chiasma. The pituitary stalk is connected with the hypothalamus, the part of the brain concerned with emotion, sleep, appetite and salt regulation, itself producing hormones which stimulate or inhibit the release of pituitary hormones.

The pituitary gland has two parts: anterior and posterior.

(a) DISORDERS OF ANTERIOR PITUITARY

Growth hormone deficiency may arise from tumour or spontaneously, and causes shortness of stature in children.

Acromegaly

Excessive production of growth hormone causes gigantism if it occurs before the epiphyses of the bones have united. In adults, it results in acromegaly. This literally means enlargement of distal tissues – hands and feet, and also the lower jaw which becomes prominent, with coarsening of the facial features. Some cases are due to tumour and the optic chiasma may also be involved, causing visual field defects. Diabetes may also be associated, as HGH is diabetogenic.

Lack of pituitary gonadotrophins causes amenorrhoea and infertility. Lack of the gonadal hormones secondary to gonadotrophin deficiency causes loss of sexual characteristics, and the skin becomes fine and excessively wrinkled.

Under-activity of the anterior pituitary

Causes

This may occur after post-partum haemorrhage, but may also

arise spontaneously, or as a result of tumour or infiltration of the anterior pituitary gland.

Symptoms and signs

There is commonly a history of failure to lactate after pregnancy.

The periods do not return.

Sexual hair disappears.

The skin is pale yet the patient is not anaemic.

The patient is weak and hypotensive from lack of cortisol, and there is a varying degree of hypothyroidism.

Investigations

The diagnosis is confirmed by finding low blood levels of cortisol and thyroxine. Tests of the 'pituitary–adrenal axis' help to localize the fault in the anterior pituitary. These include response to ACTH, and insulin hypoglycaemia.

(b) DISORDERS OF THE POSTERIOR PITUITARY

The posterior pituitary releases the antidiuretic hormone (ADH, vasopressin) in response to a signal from an area of the hypothalamus sensitive to increased tonicity (osmolality) of the blood. ADH acts on the renal tubules, causing reabsorption of water into the circulation and correcting the tonicity of the blood – and less urine is formed.

Diabetes insipidus

This is due to lack of ADH, which may follow destruction of the posterior pituitary by tumour, trauma, or infection (such as encephalitis).

Symptoms and signs

The patient passes large quantities of extremely dilute urine – specific gravity around 1000 – just like water.

There is great thirst and if fluid is withheld the patient will go to any extreme to obtain water.

DIFFERENTIAL DIAGNOSIS – OF SPECIFIC ENDOCRINE PROBLEMS

	Onset	*Pre-existing conditions*
Diabetes (maturity onset)	slow, gradual	middle-aged or elderly (mostly female); family history sometimes; lethargy
Diabetes (juvenile growth onset)	rapid, may proceed to coma	coryza or other bacterial virus infection, predominantly in young or adolescent; strong family history; fatigue progressive, drastic weight loss, ketoacidosis
Hyperthyroidism (thyrotoxicosis)	may develop quickly or progressively	commoner in women, loss of weight, may be exophthalmos; thyroid gland may be enlarged
Hypothyroidism (myxoedema)	slow	commonest in middle-aged women; lethargy; may have goitre; intolerance to cold; may have dyspnoea or dysphagia, depending on size of goitre
Hyperadrenalism (Cushing's disease)	slow	obesity, 'moon face', muscular weakness, plethora, lassitude; some recent weight loss
Hypoadrenalism (Addison's disease)	insidious but may be acute	weight loss, weakness, fatigue, anorexia; may follow previous illness, sepsis or haemorrhage
Hyperpituitarism	slow, particularly during growth period	gigantism if during growth period, acromegaly in adult; visual field defects
Hypopituitarism	slow, may be rapid following other illness	may have been severe illness or post-partum haemorrhage; fatigue, depression, failure to lactate; weight loss

Associated findings	*Key laboratory findings*
obesity, polyuria, vascular disease, pruritis	raised random blood sugar, glycosuria, abnormal glucose tolerance test; hyperlipaemia
polyuria, drowsiness, vomiting, air-hunger, dehydration	glycosuria, acetonuria, blood sugar high (fasting in excess of 180 mg/100 ml, 10 mmol/l)
rapid pulse even sleeping; 'bruit' audible over gland; hyperactivity	raised T_4 and uptake of ^{131}I; thyroxine levels high; lymphocytosis
depression, loss of hair, coarsening of facial features	low serum thyroxine, raised TSH response, hypercholesterolaemia; thyroglobin antibodies
amenorrhoea, virilism, hypertension, osteoporosis, may be diabetes; specific cutaneous pigmentation	raised urinary and serum cortisol; raised ACTH anaemia, hypokalaemia; X-ray skull may show pituitary fossa changes
low blood pressure, brown skin pigmentation in flexures and 'tanned' in both exposed and unexposed parts	serum Na low, K and urea raised; low plasma cortisol; X-ray of chest may show diminished cardiac size; intravenous ACTH test abnormal
amenorrhoea, infertility, loss of libido, skin changes; headache	high growth hormone levels and low serum sex hormones; may be diabetic in response to GTT
amenorrhoea, loss of pubic hair; hypotension; may have diabetes insipidus if post-pituitary involved	low serum cortisol and thyroxine; hypoglycaemia; polyuria, polydipsia

Chapter 12
The Nutritional System and Acid–Base Balance

The commonest disorder of nutrition in the developed world is obesity due to excessive food intake, and it is now held to affect one in five of the population. In the rest of the world it is malnutrition due to an insufficient supply of food. Vitamin deficiency is, however, seen in all localities due to poverty and is, in some areas, becoming particularly more common in the elderly. In hospital, deficiencies and disorders due to problems with body water, electrolyte and acid–base balance in those patients on treatment, is of increasing importance.

Diagnosis of disorder will depend on symptoms, history, observation of the patient and examination of:

(A) body weight,
(B) blood tests,
(C) X-rays,
(D) urine tests,
(E) fluid input–output measurement.

Common symptoms of generalized disorder will be:

(1) fatigue, weakness and malaise,
(2) breathlessness (exertional),
(3) skin rashes,
(4) oedema,
(5) anaemia,
(6) growth deficiency,
(7) orthopaedic disorders (e.g. osteoporosis/arthritis).

(A) BODY WEIGHT

A patient is considered overweight if weighing over 20 lb (8 kg) more than the norm for age, sex, height and body build. Tables (see page 61) published by life insurance companies offer guides for adult norms. Fat normally constitutes 20% of total body weight, and skinfold thickness can also be assessed (greater than 23 mm, male; or 30 mm female, over the triceps in the upper arm). The diagnosis of obesity or gross undernutrition is, however, frequently obvious in the initial assessment of the patient's physique.

(B) BLOOD TESTS

In vitamin deficiency and malnutrition anaemia is common. Full blood film, count and serum assessments will be necessary. In acid–base balance monitoring blood gases, arterial and venous tests are necessary, as well as the electrolyte status.

(C) X-RAYS

Osteoporosis or osteomalacia is assessed by X-ray, as is age in the underdeveloped or malnourished child, by defining ossification centre activity.

(D) URINE TESTS

Saturation tests for vitamin C absorption, or the detection of excess calcium salts, may be employed. Urine measurement and output and its concentration (specific gravity) in maintaining acid–base balance, is essential. Urea and acetone content of urine in starvation is a useful guide to diagnosis.

(E) FLUID INPUT–OUTPUT CHARTS

In all patients given i.v. fluids, for trauma, surgery or correction of deficiency, the most scrupulous recording and measurement of what is received, what is taken orally, and what is excreted is necessary. The input–output chart is of as much importance to patient therapy as the confirmatory serum assessments.

Common Disorders of Nutrition

(1) OBESITY

(a) Most commonly caused by overeating – either an excessive calorie intake or excessive dependence on carbohydrate foodstuffs in the diet.

(b) *Genetic and environmental.* Obesity can start in childhood and there may be a genetic basis in some children who have inherited a greater number of adipose tissue cells than others. However, children tend to follow the eating habits of their parents. Thus obesity often runs in families.

(c) *Disturbed calorie balance.* Obese people often claim to eat no more than their thinner fellows. Again, some people eat a lot yet do not become fat. As the muscles of the obese are not more efficient in their use of calories than those of the thin, the explanation must lie in different energy expenditure or heat loss. Thin people increase their metabolic rate in response to food consumption, channelling the glucose to be utilized in muscle activity. Fat people may fail to do this, for in association with an increased insulin production characteristic of obesity, their glucose is directed towards the fat depots instead. They may be unable to generate as much heat as their thinner colleagues, having a thermogenic defect related to their 'brown adipose tissue'. Lean people have a higher metabolic response to adrenaline-like drugs. The obese are generally less active and take less exercise than thin people – exercise and weight loss may help to correct the metabolic abnormalities of obesity.

Thus obesity may be due to inadequate exercise in a modern society where physical activity at work is no longer required, because of the use of machinery, and even the benefits of walking to work have been removed by buses, cars and trains. The gradual onset of obesity in middle age is usually due to decreased energy expenditure with an unchanged calorie intake.

(d) *Endocrine.* The obesity of Cushing's syndrome affects only the trunk, the arms and legs being thin, and the skin is thinned. The obese rarely have overt evidence of 'glandular disturbance', but as obesity often follows childbirth or the menopause, endocrine factors play a part, possibly through effects on hypothalamic control.

(e) *Psychological.* There does not seem to be a particularly high incidence of psychiatric disturbance in obese people attending hospitals. A proportion may be of tense and anxious disposition and they gain solace from their worries by overeating.

EFFECTS

Cardiovascular

There is a raised incidence of hypertension and arteriosclerotic disease, especially ischaemic heart disease – the mechanical burden on the heart and altered blood fats are responsible. Strokes and renal failure are commoner in the obese. Varicose veins, thromboembolism and pulmonary infarction are complications.

Respiratory

The layers of fat impede ventilation, with increased tendency to bronchitis and pneumonia, or chronic anoxia in extreme cases.

Joints and ligaments

Backache, arthritis – especially of the knees and hips.

Metabolic

Increased incidence of diabetes, the insulin produced being

ultimately unable to cope with the demands of the great bulk of fatty tissue. Increased tendency to gallstones and cholecystitis from cholesterol upset.

Surgical problems
Access at operations is difficult, wound healing is impaired with risk of incisional hernia, and post-operative pneumonia and pulmonary infarction are commoner in the obese.

Life-expectancy
The obese have a shortened life-expectancy and, when ill, a mortality rate some 30% greater than that of the non-obese suffering from the same condition.

(2) VITAMIN DEFICIENCY

A normal mixed diet provides adequate vitamins. Deficiency can occur from:
(1) dietary lack – infants, the elderly, alcoholics and food fads;
(2) failure of absorption – malabsorption syndrome, gastric surgery;
(3) effects of drugs – such as folic acid deficiency due to anti-convulsants.

(a) VITAMIN A (RETINOL)

Vitamin A is found in animal fats and dairy products, fish liver oils and as a provitamin in carrots and tomatoes. It is concerned in copper metabolism, is necessary for the formation of visual purple in the retina and for the maintenance of epithelial tissues including the skin and cornea.

Deficiency: causes night blindness; a serious deficiency causes degeneration of the cornea.

(b) VITAMIN B COMPLEX

This includes vitamin B_1 (aneurine, thiamine), vitamin B_2 (riboflavine), pyridoxine or vitamin B_6, and nicotinic acid (nicotinamide, vitamin B_7), vitamin B_{12} and folic acid.

Vitamins of B complex are found in meat, eggs and dairy produce (milk is a rich source of riboflavine), and cereal germ and bran (rich in aneurine). The vitamins form part of enzyme systems concerned in carbohydrate metabolism. Vitamin B_1 is added to white bread.

Deficiency: isolated vitamin B_1 deficiency causes wet beri-beri – cardiac failure with oedema and warm extremities, and neurological upset. This includes encephalopathy, cerebral beri-beri – a confusional state plus signs of brain-stem involvement such as nystagmus and ocular nerve palsies. Nutritional peripheral neuritis, dry beri-beri, occurs in alcoholics and after long illnesses associated with vomiting and poor dietary intake.

Vitamin B_2 deficiency may occur in malabsorption states and causes cracks at the corners of the mouth (angular cheilitis) and sore, red tongue. Such findings also occur in nicotinic acid deficiency, which classically causes pellagra – dermatitis, diarrhoea and dementia.

Findings such as a sore tongue or cracked lips should indicate the possibility of vitamin B deficiency in alcoholics or the elderly.

Pyridoxine deficiency may complicate isoniazid therapy for tuberculosis due to metabolic interference, causing peripheral neuritis; deficiency may also cause the rare sideroblastic anaemia.

(c) VITAMIN B_{12}

This is found in liver, meat, eggs and milk.

Deficiency: extremely rare, occurring only in Vegans, a strict vegetarian sect who eat no animal protein whatsoever. Pernicious anaemia is due to lack of vitamin B_{12} from malabsorption following gastric atrophy and lack of intrinsic factor, and malabsorption can also occur after gastric surgery.

(d) FOLIC ACID

This is found in liver and green vegetables, but may be destroyed in cooking.

Deficiency: may occur in the elderly, needs are increased in pregnancy; malabsorption may occur in intestinal disease, and anticonvulsant drugs impair its availability for metabolism. The result is a macrocytic anaemia, and possibly dementia in the elderly. Pregnant women are given supplements of 100 µg (plus iron) to prevent deficiency.

(e) VITAMIN C (ASCORBIC ACID)

Ascorbic acid is found in fruits (e.g. blackcurrants), rose hips, tomatoes and green vegetables. Potatoes contain some vitamin C and as they are a staple article of Western diet they provide a considerable part of the daily requirement. Stored potatoes lack the vitamin, so deficiency may be seen in winter and spring before the new crop is available. Elderly people may take little fruit and vegetables, subsisting on tea and toast. In hospital they are still at risk from vitamin C deficiency, for high temperatures and bulk cooking destroy it, and hospital food may be deficient. Babies are born with a sufficient reserve of vitamin C for some months and breast milk contains the vitamin. There is little in cows' milk and it is destroyed by pasteurization.

Deficiency: results in scurvy – purpuric haemorrhages into the skin and mucous membranes. The legs are especially affected; other signs are scaliness of the skin around the hair follicles. There is bleeding from the gums (and from under the periosteum of the bones in infants), anaemia and general debility. Wounds are slow to heal.

(f) VITAMIN D

Natural vitamin D is vitamin D_3, cholecalciferol, found in animal fat and formed in the skin by the action of ultraviolet light. Ultraviolet radiation of certain plant substances produces the synthetic vitamin D_2, calciferol, which has the same action. Butter, cheese, egg-yolk and fish-liver oils are good sources of vitamin D. Margarine is fortified with calciferol.

Vitamin D is hydroxylated in the liver and again in the kidney to its most active form, calcitriol. Vitamin D promotes the absorption of calcium and phosphate from the gut and has a direct action on bone, causing laying down of calcium salt on the protein matrix – mineralization. Requirements are greatest in childhood, pregnancy, and lactation; recommended daily intake 400 units (10 ug). Blood levels of hydroxy-vitamin D can be measured.

Causes of deficiency

(1) *Dietary lack* in infants, and in the elderly.
(2) *Malabsorption*: the vitamin is fat-soluble and requires the presence of bile salts for emulsification. Malabsorption occurs in biliary cirrhosis and other malabsorption syndromes.
(3) *Lack of sunshine*: atmospheric pollution screens off the sun's ultraviolet rays and, since pigmented skin is less sensitive to ultraviolet than fair skin, deficiency of vitamin D has occurred in the infants of coloured immigrants living in temperate or urban environments.
(4) *Chronic renal disease*: failure of conversion of vitamin D to its active form.

Results of deficiency: rickets and osteomalacia

Deficiency results in rickets in children – defective calcification of the bones with swelling of the tissue at their growing ends, impaired growth, and softening of the shafts causing deformities such as bowing of the legs. There is muscle weakness, abdominal distension and tetany from the low blood calcium.

Vitamin D deficiency in adults results in osteomalacia, demineralization and rarefaction of the bones. There are bone pains, and trivial injury may result in fractures of the long bones; tiny symptomless fractures may be seen on X-ray of the pelvis, which may become grossly deformed later. There is muscular weakness and a waddling gait. Osteomalacia may occur in the elderly.

(g) VITAMIN E

This is contained in wheat-germ oil.

Deficiency: causes infertility in rats but this is not known to occur in human deficiency.

(h) VITAMIN K

Vitamin K was originally found in pig-liver fat but it is also present in the leaves of plants such as spinach and cabbage, and in many vegetable oils. In addition, it is manufactured by bacteria in the gut. The naturally occurring forms are vitamins K_1 and K_2 which are non-toxic even when given in big doses.

Vitamin K is necessary for the production of prothrombin and other clotting factors by the liver.

Deficiency: is unknown, but malabsorption of the vitamin occurs in obstructive jaundice from lack of bile salts, and in conditions such as coeliac syndrome. Deficiency may rarely occur from the prolonged use of oral broad-spectrum antibiotics which alter the intestinal flora. In adults, cirrhosis of the liver impairs prothrombin production. Oral anticoagulants act by competing with vitamin K in the liver, blocking the formation of prothrombin.

Prothrombin deficiency: results in a bruising tendency, haematuria and failure of the blood to clot.

(3) MINERAL DEFICIENCIES

(a) Calcium

Milk and dairy products are rich sources of calcium. An average diet contains 1–2 g calcium daily. Only about a tenth of this is absorbed, balanced by a similar excretion in the urine. Absorption is dependent on vitamin D, and is higher in growing children where calcium is required for the bones, and in pregnant and lactating women. Absorption is also increased where there is excessive bone destruction and loss of calcium in the urine as in hyperparathyroidism, where demineralization and fractures occur if absorption does not keep pace with demand.

Hypocalcaemia, lowering of the blood calcium, occurs in hypoparathyroidism and to a lesser degree in vitamin D deficiency – rickets and osteomalacia.

States of alkalosis decrease the solubility of calcium in the blood, so that hypocalcaemic symptoms may follow prolonged vomiting with loss of hydrochloric acid, or over-breathing, which washes out carbon dioxide and carbonic acid.

Hypocalcaemia causes increased excitability of the nerves and results in tetany.

There is a numbness and tingling in fingers, toes or around the lips, and a characteristic spasm at the hands and feet – carpopedal spasm.

The wrists and metacarpophalangeal joints are held in flexion, with the fingers in extension. The sign may be provoked by pressure on the arm with a sphygmomanometer cuff.

Tapping over the facial nerve in front of the ear elicits twitching of the lips and muscles of the face.

There may be spasm of the muscles of the larynx, with prolonged 'crowing' inspiration, dyspnoea and cyanosis. Convulsions, and epileptic attacks in those predisposed to them, may be precipitated.

Prolonged hypocalcaemia causes muscle weakness, a coarse, dry skin, calcium deposits in the cornea, and raised intra-cranial pressure with convulsions or precipitation of epilepsy.

Hypercalcaemia occurs in vitamin D intoxication, hyper-parathyroidism, bone diseases such as myelomatosis, and sometimes in carcinomatosis and sarcoidosis. Symptoms include lassitude, anorexia, nausea, vomiting, polyuria, thirst and renal failure follows.

(b) Magnesium

Magnesium is required in small quantities; its actions have some similarities to those of calcium.

(c) Iron

Iron is necessary for the formation of haemoglobin. (See Chapter 13, 'The blood and lymphatic system'.)

(d) Copper

Traces are necessary for blood formation and possibly for nerve function.

(e) Iodine

Small quantities are necessary for normal thyroid function and formation of the thyroid hormone thyroxine. Deficiency is one cause of goitre, or thyroid swelling.

(f) Fluorine

A concentration of one part per million in the water supply lowers the incidence of dental caries. Excessive doses cause fluorosis, a hardening of the bones.

(4) ELECTROLYTE AND ACID–BASE BALANCE DISORDERS

The body has three sources of water – the water drunk, the water present in food, and the water formed by the metabolic oxidation of food. Water is lost in the urine, in the faeces, and by evaporation from the skin and exhaled air from the lungs. The daily balance is as follows:

Water intake		*Water output*	
Water drunk	1500 ml	Urine	1500 ml
Water in food	500–1000 ml	Faeces	100 ml
Metabolic water	200– 500 ml	Skin evaporation	500 ml
		Lungs	400 ml
TOTAL	2.5 litres	TOTAL	2.5 litres

Evaporation from the skin and exhaled air represents an obligatory litre of water per day; if the amount necessary for adequate urinary excretion is added, then basal requirements are about 2 litres daily. Much higher intakes may be required in hot climates and in fevers, when skin losses are greatly increased.

Salts such as sodium chloride when dissolved in water dissociate into particles. Thus sodium chloride dissociates into sodium (Na), and chloride (Cl). These particles are called ions and carry an electrical charge – hence the salts from which they are formed are called electrolytes. Important salts or electrolytes in the body fluids are sodium chloride, sodium bicarbonate and potassium chloride.

The strength, tonicity or osmolality of a solution depends on the total number of particles dissolved in it – the main contribution is from the electrolytes.

In general terms, water will pass from a more dilute solution on one side of a membrane to a more concentrated solution on the other in an attempt to equalize the concentration on both sides of the membrane – the concentrated solution exerts an osmotic force which attracts water. The tonicity or osmolality of the body fluids bathing the cells has to be kept constant and equal to that inside the cells, otherwise these lose or attract water, and break up or burst.

Sodium is the dominant ion responsible for the maintenance of the extracellular fluid volume – that is, for the retention of water. Potassium is the dominant intracellular ion. The cell membrane uses energy to keep sodium out of, and to keep potassium in, the cell. In the blood vessels the osmotic force exerted by the plasma proteins, especially albumin, helps to maintain the circulating fluid volume.

The volume of fluid in the body depends partly on the stimulus of a rise in tonicity affecting a centre in the hypothalamus, causing release of antidiuretic hormone and therefore water retention, and partly on special volume receptors in the circulation – these may act via the kidney regulating sodium loss. The sensation of thirst is one regulator of intake, but the control of the body fluids is largely dependent on the kidneys, which vary the excretion of water and salts to maintain normality.

(a) ELECTROLYTE BALANCE

Under basal conditions very little dietary salt (sodium chloride) is necessary, for the kidneys can, if required, secrete a urine almost free of sodium and chloride, and no salt is lost in the normal insensitive evaporation of water from the skin. Thus 1–2 g salt daily is sufficient, except where losses are great, as in visible sweating and in high fevers. Normal foods contain little sodium, but man has developed a taste for salt, preserved and canned meats and sausages containing large amounts. Thus the dietary intake is very variable, from 5 g to 20 g daily of sodium chloride, averaging 12 g which corresponds to 160 mmol sodium. This is usually much in excess of needs, the kidneys excreting the excess.

The kidneys cannot conserve potassium – there is an obligatory daily loss in the urine (unlike sodium). Animal and plant cells are rich in potassium and therefore most natural foods contain it – fruit juices are a rich source. The normal potassium intake is about 6 g potassium chloride, equivalent to 70 mmol potassium, daily.

Sampling the blood gives an indication of the fluid and electrolyte balance of the patient – the packed cell volume (haematocrit), sodium, potassium and chloride being easily estimated.

(b) ACID–BASE BALANCE

Tissue respiration results in the production of carbon dioxide, which is duly excreted by the lung. Exercise, protein and fat breakdown also result in the production of acids. Thus metabolic processes are acid-forming.

The acidity of a solution is commonly expressed on the pH scale. It should be understood that a very small change in pH represents a big difference in concentration. Chemical neutrality is pH 7, the pH of water. Acids have a pH lower than 7, alkalis a pH higher than 7. The pH of plasma has to be maintained at 7.4, just on the alkaline side. Metabolic processes would tend to shift the pH downwards, the state of acidosis. This tendency is resisted by the presence of 'buffer systems' in the blood which bind acids harmlessly until they can be excreted as carbon dioxide by the lungs, or by the kidney tubules. An important and readily measurable buffer system is the bicarbonate system. Not only do the kidneys excrete acids, they also reconstitute bicarbonate buffer and return it to the bloodstream. While the urinary pH is a guide to the acidic concentration in the body if the kidneys are working normally, blood measurements are more accurate and are an essential part of the management of acid–base disturbances.

A tendency for the pH to fall, that is, a state of acidosis, is recognized by a fall in the plasma bicarbonate ('buffer base deficit'), or a rise in the carbon dioxide. The former occurs in diabetic ketoacidosis and renal failure, the latter in the respiratory acidosis of respiratory failure.

For the preservation of a normal acid–base balance, the body needs a sufficient supply of water and electrolytes, a normal cardiac output, and adequately functioning lungs and kidneys.

Disturbances of Water and Electrolyte Balance

(a) WATER DEFICIENCY

A deficiency purely of water is usually due to insufficient intake – in desert conditions, inability to swallow, or in comas. Water deficiency can also follow urinary losses in diabetes.

As a result, the tonicity of the extracellular fluid tends to rise, and water moves out from the cells into the extracellular fluid. The intracellular dehydration causes the symptom of thirst in the conscious patient, the tongue is dry, and the urine decreased in amount but very concentrated, of high specific gravity.

(b) PURE SALT DEPLETION

Salt losses occur with severe sweating in the tropics and in men doing heavy manual work in hot conditions such as foundries. Symptoms include muscle cramps and weakness. In pure salt depletion the sodium concentration in the plasma falls and the urine flow might be increased to maintain it. This results in water passing from the circulation into the cells to equalize the osmotic pressure. Thus there is a lack of fluid in circulation and a fall in blood pressure, but as there is cellular overhydration the patient is not thirsty.

In clinical practice pure water or salt deficiency states are rare – usually the deficiency is a combined one, giving the picture called dehydration.

(c) THE CLINICAL PICTURE OF DEHYDRATION

The clinical state of dehydration is a result of water and salt deficiency, usually from abnormal losses. The extracellular fluid becomes depleted but for a time plasma volume can be maintained. Once the deficiency has reached several litres, the blood volume is reduced and the circulation to the kidneys impaired, leading to acidosis and uraemia.

Causes

Insufficient intake of fluids as in coma or, more commonly, excessive losses of fluids from the body.

Severe vomiting and diarrhoea; also paralytic ileus, a complication of intestinal obstruction of operation when fluid is poured into the gut and lost to the circulation.

Sweating, especially in fevers in hot climates.

Polyuria in diabetes mellitus or chronic renal failure.

Severe burns – loss of serum from skin damage.

Severe haemorrhage produces pallor and collapse, a different picture, but dehydration may be a complication, especially in haematemesis.

Symptoms and signs

Thirst is usual, but may be absent if the deficiency is mainly of salt.

Patient weak and lethargic.

Tongue dry.

Skin inelastic and slack, remaining in a fold when pinched up.

The eyes may be sunken.

The pulse rises, blood pressure falls.

Coma may result.

Output of urine is markedly reduced, it is concentrated (high specific gravity) if the kidneys are healthy.

With renal failure and acidosis, there is vomiting and deep sighing respirations – acidotic breathing, air hunger.

Observations and investigations

The nature and extent of the fluid loss, and the urine volume must be noted – an input–output chart must be kept, plus record of pulse, blood pressure and weight if possible.

Urine tests include specific gravity, urea and sodium concentration.

Haemoglobin and haematocrit are raised in dehydration and the blood urea may be raised. The sodium and other electrolyte levels are a guide to therapy.

(d) OVER-HYDRATION

In health, it is almost impossible to drink too much fluid – the kidneys will excrete the excess. Over-hydration results from excessive intravenous fluids, especially in patients with poor circulation and failing kidneys.

Symptoms and signs

Include lethargy, anorexia and vomiting.

Venous pressure is raised, and jugular venous pulsation may be seen in the neck.

Fluid accumulates in the lungs, causing breathlessness and crepitations ('moist' sounds heard with the stethoscope over the lung bases).

Peripheral oedema develops.

Hypertension, especially in association with renal failure.

(e) OEDEMA

Oedema is due to the accumulation of excess fluid in the interstitial space.

Causes

Local

(1) Increased permeability of small blood vessels as in trauma, burns, inflammation and infection, and allergy (angioneurotic oedema).
(2) Lymphatic obstruction – in carcinoma and in tropical filariasis.
(3) Venous obstruction – thrombosis, pressure of tumours.

Generalized

(1) *Cardiac failure* due to an excess of fluid both in the circulation and in the tissues. Deranged volume receptors in the circulation may act through antidiuretic hormone secretion to cause water retention by the kidneys; in addition, a reduced renal blood flow results in sodium retention, and aldosterone secretion may worsen this. Thus there is salt and water retention.

    In cardiac failure the additional factor of the raised venous pressure aggravates oedema formation in dependent regions.
(2) *Hypoproteinaemic states*:
    nephrotic syndrome,
    cirrhosis of the liver,
    malnutrition ('famine oedema'),
    severe malabsorption.

    In these conditions the plasma protein, especially albumin, is lowered. This results in lowered plasma osmotic pressure, the force which attracts water into solution. When it is lowered, water passes from the blood vessels into the tissues. The tendency for the circulating blood volume to fall causes excess aldosterone secretion which acts on the renal tubules to cause salt and water retention, worsening the tissue oedema.
(3) *Acute glomerulonephritis.* The puffiness of the face and peripheral oedema results from sodium and water retention related to the renal disorder.
(4) *Toxaemia of pregnancy* (oedema, albuminuria, hypertension and fits) has a similar basis.
(5) *Corticosteroid (e.g. cortisone) overdosage*, and sometimes in Cushing's syndrome.

Clinical presentation of oedema

There is swelling on the affected part, and the skin 'pits' on pressure with the fingertip due to the subcutaneous fluid.

Oedema accumulates in the dependent parts of the body and where the skin is lax, ankle swelling is often the first sign.

Breathlessness from pulmonary oedema.

In the hypoproteinaemic states such as nephrotic syndrome, and in acute glomerulonephritis, the patient can lie flat without discomfort, so oedema may gather about the face, hands and arms.

Effusions occur into the pleural and peritoneal cavities.

Ascites where there is a raised portal venous pressure.

(f) DISTURBANCES OF POTASSIUM BALANCE

HYPOKALAEMIA

Abnormally low serum potassium, indicates that a severe degree of intracellular depletion has occurred.

Causes

Loss from gastrointestinal tract, especially diarrhoea, in diseases such as cholera and severe ulcerative colitis; also abuse of purgatives.

Renal losses and polyuria resulting from:
- prolonged use of diuretics;
- polyuria following acute renal failure;
- use of forced diuretic therapy in aspirin poisoning.

Cardiac failure.

Cirrhosis. Potassium loss is associated with disturbed cell function, and will be worsened by diuretic therapy unless supplements are given.

Diabetic ketoacidosis – loss from the cells and into the urine has occurred and in the recovery stages blood levels of potassium may be low.

Excess aldosterone secretion and after prolonged use of corticosteroids.

Symptoms and signs

Apathy, fatigue, confusion, muscle weakness.

Intestinal slowing and ileus (paralysis) with abdominal distension.

Polyuria.

ECG changes, due to cardiac arrhythmias such as extrasystoles.

HYPERKALAEMIA

Excessive potassium in the blood (normal serum potassium is 4.25 mmol/l) but it need not indicate a high intracellular level.

Causes

Renal failure is the commonest cause of failure to excrete potassium. In acute renal failure there is oliguria and as the causative condition is usually associated with tissue damage and release of potassium from the cells, the level in the blood rises rapidly. In chronic renal failure the kidneys may excrete potassium normally until the late stages, when hyperkalaemia occurs.

Poor renal function and cellular breakdown cause hyperkalaemia in some cases of diabetic ketoacidosis, and states of circulatory failure and anoxia.

The serum potassium level is raised in Addison's disease from cortisol (hydrocortisone) lack, but the sodium deficiency is more important.

Symptoms and signs

Muscle weakness.

ECG changes (tall T waves).

When the serum potassium reaches 7 mmol/l, there is a danger of asystole and cardiac arrest.

(g) DISTURBANCE OF ACID–BASE BALANCE

ACIDOSIS

This is a tendency for the blood to become more acid, or rather less alkaline, than normal. The pH is lowered from its normal 7.4 but seldom falls below 7.2. The body has two routes for getting rid of acids – the lungs losing carbon dioxide and the kidneys excreting; the kidneys also reconstitute bicarbonate, returning it to the circulation.

Acidosis is classified as (a) *respiratory* or (b) *non-respiratory.* (a) Respiratory acidosis is due to impaired excretion of CO_2 in respiratory failure – in conditions such as chronic bronchitis and emphysema with superadded infection, and less commonly in the respiratory depression of poisoning, or following respiratory muscle paralysis (in these states anoxia is more dominant). Thus the CO_2 dissolved in the blood, $P\text{CO}_2$, is raised above the normal 40 mmHg (5.3 kPa), the condition called hypercapnia.

The causative condition is usually associated with dyspnoea and cyanosis from anoxia, and the CO_2 retention contributes to the restlessness, confusion, disturbance of consciousness, and tremor.

Causes

Diabetic ketoacidosis – the ketone bodies are themselves acids.

Renal failure.

Conditions such as renal tubular acidosis, and ureteric implantation into the colon which may impair renal tubular function.

Conditions associated with water and salt depletion impairing renal function, such as prolonged vomiting or diarrhoea with loss of intestinal secretions including bicarbonate, or high fevers with lack of fluid intake; i.e. clinical dehydration.

Cardiac arrest and circulatory failure.

Symptoms and signs

Lethargy and weakness.

Vomiting.

The raised concentration stimulates the respiratory centre causing deep sighing respiration or 'air hunger' in an attempt to get rid of the excess acids as carbon dioxide from the lungs.

Finally, the patient lapses into unconsciousness.

Investigations

Investigations include the blood pH and bicarbonate, which are lowered: there is a 'base deficit'. Haemoglobin, haematocrit, urea, sugar and electrolytes are also measured, and $P\text{CO}_2$.

ALKALOSIS

The blood is too alkaline, with a rise in pH. Alkalosis is not common but may be respiratory or non-respiratory.

Causes

Respiratory alkalosis

Over-breathing with loss of CO_2 and carbonic acid.

Overbreathing occurs in anxiety, hysteria and occasionally following damage to the respiratory centre in the brain stem.

In the early stages of aspirin poisoning, overbreathing is due to stimulation of the respiratory centre by the salicylate.

Non-respiratory alkalosis

Prolonged vomiting or aspiration of gastric contents, with loss of hydrochloric acid, as may occur in pyloric stenosis.

Excessive intake of alkalis such as sodium bicarbonate, taken to relieve the pain of peptic ulcer.

A consequence of potassium depletion.

Symptoms and signs

Decreases the amount of calcium in the blood, causing increased excitability of the nerves and muscles.

Paraesthesiae (tingling feelings, pins and needles).

Clouding of consciousness and convulsions.

DIFFERENTIAL DIAGNOSIS OF VITAMIN DEFICIENCY

	Sources
Vitamin A	animal fats, dairy produce, fish-liver oils
Vitamin B complex	meat, eggs, dairy produce, cereal germ, bran
Vitamin B_{12}	liver, meat, eggs, milk
Folic acid	liver, green vegetables
Vitamin C	fruits (esp. blackcurrants), green vegetables, rose hips
Vitamin D	animal fats, fish oils, dairy produce
Vitamin E	wheat-germ oil
Vitamin K	pork liver, spinach, cabbage; vegetable oils

Signs of deficiency	*Key laboratory findings*
night vision defects, corneal degeneration	serum tocopherol level lowered
beri-beri, neuropathies, cheilitis, glossitis, anaemia	serum levels lowered; FBC abnormalities
pernicious anaemia	FBC abnormalities; serum levels lowered; bone marrow changes
macrocytic anaemia	FBC abnormalities; serum levels lowered; bone marrow changes
scurvy, purpura, gingivitis, anaemia, debility, reduced wound healing	WBC ascorbate level lowered; saturation test response (urine)
rickets in children, osteomalacia, muscular weakness	serum calcium levels altered; X-ray changes at epiphyses; serum levels altered
none recognized	none recognized
prothrombin deficiency, clotting mechanism interference	prothrombin levels altered; bleeding time extended

DIFFERENTIAL DIAGNOSIS OF ELECTROLYTE AND ACID–BASE BALANCE DISTURBANCE

	Causes
Acidosis	respiratory, due to failure, chronic bronchitis, emphysema, dyspnoea and cyanosis diabetic ketoacidosis renal failure prolonged vomiting, diarrhoea dehydration cardiac arrest, circulatory failure
Alkalosis	respiratory due to hyperventilation salicylate poisoning prolonged vomiting excessive oral intake alkalis potassium depletion
Hypokalaemia	losses from GIT, e.g. severe and continual diarrhoea excess diuresis renal, cardiac, liver failure diabetic ketoacidosis
Hyperkalaemia	renal failure and oliguria hypoadrenalism (Addison's disease) circulatory failure and anoxia excessive intake

Symptoms and signs	*Key laboratory findings*
lethargy, vomiting, deep sighing respiration – tremor, restlessness, confusion; coma	lowered blood pH and plasma bicarbonate; high $P\text{CO}_2$
increased muscular and nervous excitability, paraesthesia, confusion, 'tetany', convulsions	raised blood pH; raised plasma bicarbonate; lowered $P\text{CO}_2$
anorexia, nausea, fatigue, confusion, polyuria, intestinal ileus, cardiac (ECG) arrhythmias	serum potassium lowered; urine potassium level lowered over 24 h if renal in origin
muscle weakness, irritability, confusion, ECG changes – asystole and cardiac arrest	serum potassium raised

Tetany includes spasm of the fingers and muscles of the larynx, and twitching of the face.

Investigations

The diagnosis is confirmed by the clinical history and tests such as plasma bicarbonate and pH, and $P\text{CO}_2$.

Chapter 13
The Blood and Lymphatic System

The commonest disorder of the blood and lymphatic system is, globally, anaemia. Even in the developed world where, in general, nutritional standards are high, as many as 15% of the population suffer iron-deficiency anaemia. Anaemias due to other deficiencies are the next most common disorder with haemorrhagic diseases and the leukaemias following. These latter, and the malignant diseases of the lymphoreticular system, are the main cause of death from disorders of this system.

Diagnosis of disorder will depend on symptoms, history, observation of the patient and examination of:

(A) blood – red cells, white cells and serum,
(B) bone marrow and biopsy.

Common symptoms of generalized disorder will be:
(1) pallor,
(2) fatigue, malaise,
(3) breathlessness,

(4) enlargement of the spleen and lymph glands,
(5) haemorrhages and bruising under the skin (purpura).

(A) EXAMINATION OF THE BLOOD

Blood consists of red cells, white cells and platelets suspended in the plasma.

Red cells (erythrocytes, RBCs) are formed in the bone marrow and contain haemoglobin, the red pigment which carries oxygen to the tissues and removes carbon dioxide. The normal haemoglobin is 100% (15 g/dl), the red cell count is 5.0×10^{12}/l (5 000 000/mm^3). Other indices include packed cell volume (PCV, normal 45%), mean cell volume (MCV) and mean corpuscular haemoglobin (MCH).

The red cell has a life of 120 days, when it is taken up and destroyed by cells of the reticuloendothelial system in the lymph glands, spleen and liver. The iron content of the 'haem' is re-utilized for blood formation, the remainder goes to form bilirubin (which becomes bile pigment), and the globin part of the haemoglobin joins the body's protein pool.

White cells (leukocytes) are of three types:

(a) Polymorphonuclear ('many-shaped nuclei') leukocytes (polymorphs, granulocytes): formed in the bone marrow, concerned in the inflammatory reaction, and in the destruction of bacteria in infections forming pus cells. The polymorphs are subdivided into neutrophils, basophils and eosinophils by the staining properties of their granules with dyes.
(b) Lymphocytes: formed in marrow, passing to lymph glands, and are of two main groups: B-lymphocytes, producing immune globulins (antibodies) and T-lymphocytes, dependent on the thymus and concerned with tissue or cellular immunity.
(c) Monocytes: fewer in number but, like the polymorphs, phagocytic in function (engulfing foreign matter).

The total white cell count (WBC) is 4.0–9.0 $\times$ 10^9/l (4000–9000/mm^3).

Platelets (thrombocytes) are produced in the bone marrow and are concerned in blood clotting.

Plasma contains water and electrolytes (e.g. sodium, potassium, chloride and bicarbonate) concerned in normal tonicity and acid–base balance and the plasma proteins, albumin, globulins, fibrinogen and prothrombin. Albumin (formed in the liver) helps to maintain the osmotic pressure, keeping fluid in the circulation. The globulins include the immune globulins, some of which are antibodies. Fibrinogen and prothrombin are concerned in blood clotting by the formation of fibrin. Blood also contains a 'fibrinolytic' mechanism to prevent excessive deposition of fibrin.

Investigations in blood disease

Minimum investigations are haemoglobin, white cell count, and erythrocyte sedimentation rate (ESR).

It is usually necessary also to stain and microscopically examine a blood film.

The plasma proteins are measured chemically, and by a method called electrophoresis, on a paper strip, or immunologically.

Serum iron or ferritin, vitamin B_{12} and folic acid levels in the blood may also be measured.

Sternal marrow puncture, using a special hollow needle (local anaesthesia) and biopsy of enlarged glands may be indicated.

(1) ANAEMIA

Anaemia is a reduction in the number of red cells, or their haemoglobin content, or both.

General symptoms and signs of anaemia

Any system may be affected.

Cardiorespiratory symptoms are breathlessness, ankle oedema and sometimes angina.

In the nervous system, effects include tiredness and faint feelings. Peripheral neuritis, leg pains and loss of reflexes may complicate any form of anaemia (but are commonest in pernicious anaemia).

In the gastrointestinal system, symptoms include loss of appetite, constipation or sometimes diarrhoea.

The characteristic sign is pallor – this may be noted classically in the conjunctivae, but pallor of the fingers and hands may also be seen.

ANAEMIA DUE TO BLOOD LOSS

The blood loss may be acute or chronic. (Chronic blood loss is the most important cause of 'iron-deficiency anaemia'.)

Acute blood loss may be obvious in injuries and gastrointestinal bleeding such as haematemesis, but less obvious with closed fractures or intra-abdominal conditions such as ruptured spleen, or retroperitoneal haemorrhage complicating anticoagulant treatment.

Symptoms and signs

Pallor.

Clammy skin.

Apprehension.

Fast pulse and low blood pressure – the picture of haemorrhagic shock, requiring transfusion.

The body compensates for such haemorrhage by haemodilution causing a temporary anaemia until the red cells have been replaced by the activity of the bone marrow, given sufficient iron.

Chronic blood loss and iron deficiency anaemia

The normal dietary iron content is 10–15 mg daily, meat and vegetable foods being rich sources. Though only a proportion of this food iron can be absorbed, it is more than enough to compensate for the daily iron losses in men, about 1–2 mg.

Thus, men rarely get 'iron deficiency' anaemia from dietary inadequacy. In women, due to menstrual blood loss, the need for iron is greater and the demand is increased by pregnancy and childbirth. The diets of many women do not meet these needs and 'iron deficiency' anaemia will ensue.

Causes of iron deficiency anaemia

(i) Blood loss: heavy menstrual bleeding (menorrhagia); chronic aspirin ingestion (causes gastric erosions); peptic ulcer; carcinoma, especially of rectum, colon or stomach; bleeds from the nose (epistaxis), and from haemorrhoids.
(ii) Increased demand – fetal needs during pregnancy.
(iii) Dietary inadequacy – occurs in women, and common in the underdeveloped world.
(iv) Defective absorption – coeliac disease; following gastrectomy or stomach operation.

Blood examination shows a low haemoglobin and some decrease in the red cell count; the cells are pale (hypochromic) and small (microcytic) – iron deficiency gives the picture described as a hypochromic, microcytic anaemia.

ANAEMIA DUE TO DECREASED BLOOD FORMATION

(a) Lack of building factors such as iron, vitamin B_{12} and folic acid. This may occur from:
    (i) inadequate dietary intake: iron deficiency is common, dietary B_{12} lack very rare, folic acid lack is rare but may occur in the elderly on a diet poor in 'greens';
    (ii) failure of absorption: pernicious anaemia;
    (iii) increased demands: anaemia of pregnancy;
    (iv) effect of anticonvulsant drugs.
(b) Lack of bone marrow – from infiltration (leukaemia), or destruction (aplastic anaemia).
(c) Disordered function of the bone marrow.

Pernicious anaemia

Cause

Pernicious anaemia has a familial tendency and is thought to be a disturbance of immunity arising in adult life. There is an autoimmune destruction of the parietal cells of the stomach, and antibodies are detectable in the circulation. The parietal cells produce hydrochloric acid and also intrinsic factor. Their destruction is followed by atrophy of the gastric mucosa, and lack of intrinsic factor. Intrinsic factor is essential for the absorption of vitamin B_{12} in the lower ileum. In pernicious anaemia, intrinsic factor is lacking and vitamin B_{12} cannot be absorbed.

Vitamin B_{12} is essential for normal bone marrow function, and in its absence red cell development is defective.

Symptoms and signs

Occurs in the middle-aged and elderly, and is commoner in women.

Onset is slow over years.

Pallor.

Low haemoglobin and often mild fever.

The skin has a lemon-yellow tint from the mild jaundice associated with haemolysis.

The tongue is smooth and often red and sore.

There is anorexia, constipation or diarrhoea.

The spleen may be palpable.

Peripheral neuritis presents as leg pains and loss of sensation, motor weakness and absent tendon reflexes (lower motor neurone lesion).

Investigations

The diagnosis is confirmed by:

(1) low haemoglobin, and the typical macrocytic blood film;
(2) megaloblastic marrow on sternal puncture;
(3) low serum vitamin B_{12};
(4) Achlorhydria: the gastric contents (obtained by tube) are found to contain no hydrochloric acid, and none is secreted after an injection of histamine.

Folic acid deficiency

Folic acid deficiency can occur from dietary lack in the elderly (from inadequate fresh vegetables) and from increased demands in pregnancy, but is usually due to malabsorption from the small intestine in tropical sprue and adult coeliac disease, gut infiltrations and following operations.

The clinical picture is similar to that in pernicious anaemia, with megaloblastic bone marrow and macrocytic peripheral blood film, but normal gastric hydrochloric acid. The serum folic acid level is low.

Anaemia from bone marrow infiltration or destruction

Anaemia in leukaemia, or in marrow infiltration by cancer metastases (such as from the breast or prostate) is due to the red cell production being replaced by abnormal proliferating cells.

Marrow destruction can be caused by X-rays (or nuclear emissions), poisons such as benzene and lead, and drugs including gold, and chloramphenicol. These may first depress platelet production (causing thrombocytopenia), or white cells (causing agranulocytosis) only later affecting red cell production, destruction of which causes aplastic anaemia.

Bone marrow function may be depressed in chronic infections and toxaemia, carcinoma and in renal failure.

INCREASED BLOOD DESTRUCTION – HAEMOLYTIC ANAEMIAS

Haemolytic anaemia may be due to defects in the red cells, or to circulating factors in the plasma which cause their destruction, or to the effects of drugs.

Faults in the red cells

Inherited

(a) Hereditary spherocytosis (congenital haemolytic anaemia, acholuric jaundice). The red cells are wrongly shaped, assuming a spherical form instead of their biconcave disc appearance. These spherocytes are fragile and haemolyse easily. The spleen is enlarged. The condition occurs mainly in children, but is rare.

(b) The haemoglobinopathies, where the haemoglobin molecule is defective.

Sickle cell disease occurs in Negro races and is common in tropical Africa and the West Indies. In affected persons, states of anoxia (from high altitudes or following infections) disturb the abnormal haemoglobin molecule causing change in shape of the red cells. They become sickle-shaped, fragile and haemolyse easily causing episodes of haemolytic anaemia.

Thalassaemia (Cooley's anaemia) occurs in Mediterranean countries and is due to a fetal type of haemoglobin persisting into adult life, the affected red cells having a 'target' appearance.

(c) Enzyme deficiencies, which increase the susceptibility of the red cells to haemolysis by substances ranging from broad beans to many drugs.

Acquired

An example is malaria, where the red cell is invaded by the *Plasmodium* parasite, causing its subsequent rupture.

Faults in the plasma

In some cases of severe pneumonia, and in carcinoma, leukaemia and renal failure, there may be circulating toxins or 'haemolysins' which destroy the red cells.

In autoimmune diseases such as systemic lupus erythematosus and rheumatoid arthritis these haemolysins may be identifiable as antibodies – immune globulins.

In certain vascular diseases and nephritis, excessive deposition of fibrin in small vessels may trap the red cells leading to their fragmentation (microangiopathic haemolytic anaemia).

Transfusing cells of the wrong group, by incompatible blood transfusion, causes the agglutinins in the plasma of the recipient to clump followed by haemolysis of the transfused cells, causing a severe reaction.

The Rhesus factor causes antibodies in a previously

sensitized mother; reaching the baby's circulation they will cause haemolysis of the fetal red cells if the baby is Rh-positive.

Effects of drugs

Many drugs are capable of causing haemolytic anaemia, especially in persons whose cells are predisposed from enzyme deficiencies, or who are already suffering from autoimmune diseases. Antimalarials and sulphonamides are common causes but chloramphenicol, nitrofurantoin, phenacetin and methyldopa may be responsible.

Symptoms and signs of haemolytic anaemia

Jaundice.

Not as deep as in obstructive jaundice.

The urine contains an excess of urobilinogen.

The spleen is enlarged and often palpable.

In severe haemolytic reactions (as may occur with incompatible blood transfusions) there are rigors, fever, prostration and often severe backache.

In very severe cases, haemoglobin is released into the bloodstream and appears, with breakdown products, in the urine, causing acute renal failure.

There is danger of 'sludging' of cells in the kidneys, causing acute renal failure.

In sickle cell disease, such sludging occurs in peripheral vessels causing pain and leg ulceration.

(2) THE HAEMORRHAGIC DISEASES

Platelet functions

The platelets can be regarded as plugging up potential holes which tend to occur in the capillary walls through wear and tear. Lack of platelets or deficiency of their 'stickiness' results in purpura and spontaneous bleeding. When a blood vessel wall is injured platelets collect at the site and liberate substances which aid vasoconstriction, thus minimizing the haemorrhage until clotting occurs.

The clotting (coagulation) mechanism has two stages:

(a) The conversion of prothrombin in the plasma to thrombin.

(b) The action of thrombin on the soluble protein fibrinogen converting it to strands of fibrin, which forms a meshwork, trapping RBCs and platelets in a clot which becomes firm by retraction.

Though platelets and calcium are involved in the first stage, only small quantities are required – even in severe deficiency of platelets, blood clotting can proceed. The many other factors needed initially include prothrombin, factor VII and anti-haemophilic globulin (factor VIII). Deficiency of any of these factors results in a clotting defect, with a prolonged 'clotting time' (normally 3–5 min).

In the second stage a deficiency of fibrinogen could prevent clotting.

Excessive deposition of fibrin in small vessels may occur in certain vascular diseases, nephritis and malignant hypertension, causing microangiopathic haemolytic anaemia.

Some of the clotting factors may be increased by the oestrogen component of the combined oestrogen–progestogen contraceptive 'pill', causing a raised incidence of venous and cerebral thrombosis in those using such tablets.

The fibrinolytic system

The clotting mechanism is balanced by the fibrinolytic mechanism which prevents intravascular thrombosis and breaks down clots that do form, by digesting fibrin.

Over-activity of the fibrinolytic system again results in the defibrination syndrome and bleeding.

Platelet aggregation is increased by cigarette smoking and by some of the prostaglandins, but inhibited by aspirin, dipyridamole and prostacyclin (generated in arterial walls).

Symptoms and signs

Spontaneous haemorrhages into the skin, mucous membranes

and internal organs. The reddish purple spots in the skin (and mouth) are called purpura, and the spots do not fade on pressure. Small purpuric spots are called petechiae, and large confluent areas are called ecchymoses which are bruise-like discolorations, occurring spontaneously.

There may be bleeding from the nose (epistaxis), mouth and alimentary tract.

There may be haematuria from renal involvement.

(Senile purpura, seen at the wrists and hands in the elderly, is due to loss of elasticity of the tissues and slight oozing of blood from shearing stresses; it is not of serious significance, and not due to capillary or platelet deficiency.)

HAEMORRHAGE DUE TO CAPILLARY DEFECT

Causes

(i) Infections: severe pneumonia, meningitis (meningococcal septicaemia), subacute bacterial endocarditis (may be embolic), haemorrhagic chickenpox and smallpox – toxaemia may be operative in these conditions.
(ii) Vitamin C (ascorbic acid) deficiency – scurvy. Occurs in elderly from lack of fruit, fresh greens or potatoes, causing blotchy haemorrhages especially on legs and thickening of the skin around the hair follicles, bleeding from the gums.
(iii) Allergic disorders – severe urticaria. Henoch–Schönlein (anaphylactoid) purpura occurs especially in children; intestinal bleeding may cause pain, melaena and precipitate intussusception (herniation of one segment of intestine into another); there are pains and swelling of the joints. Acute nephritis and renal failure may occur.
(iv) Drug sensitivity – penicillin, sulphonamides, carbromal (a hypnotic) – causing a haemorrhagic or urticarial rash.

HAEMORRHAGE DUE TO LACK OF PLATELETS — THROMBOCYTOPENIC PURPURA

Causes

(i) Poisons and drugs. The platelets are often the first to be depressed by a poison or drug affecting the bone marrow and later causing aplastic anaemia – benzene, heavy metals and gold, chloramphenicol, phenylbutazone and sulphonamides. Quinine (present in tonic water) may cause platelet antibodies to be formed.

(ii) Aplastic anaemia – often a complication of these poisons and drugs.

(iii) Leukaemia and secondary carcinomatosis of the bones – the platelets are crowded out of the marrow; severe bleeding is common in acute leukaemia.

(iv) Autoimmune diseases, such as systemic lupus erythematosus.

(v) Idiopathic thrombocytopenic purpura. The marrow is active, but platelets are not properly released.

Children may be affected, the condition in them often settling spontaneously. In young women there are recurrent episodes of purpura, spontaneous 'bruising', and they may have menorrhagia (heavy periods). In middle age, symptoms can be more severe with haemorrhage from mucous membranes and alimentary tract, haematuria and anaemia. The nurse may be the first to notice purpura at the flexure of the elbow after taking the blood pressure: the tourniquet (Hess) test utilizes a short period of venous occlusion by the sphygmomanometer cuff in suspected cases. The spleen may be enlarged, but it not necessarily palpable.

In thrombocytopenia, purpura is liable to occur when the platelet count, normal $150–350 \times 10^9/l$ ($15\,000–350\,000/mm^3$) falls below $40 \times 10^9/l$. Symptoms are severe when the level drops to $10 \times 10^9/l$ or below, and this is commonest where the thrombocytopenia is a complication of leukaemia or aplastic anaemia. At these low levels, haemorrhages may be seen in the retinae using the ophthalmoscope, and there is danger of intracranial haemorrhage, causing acute stroke or sudden death.

COAGULATION DEFECT (HAEMORRHAGE DUE TO CLOTTING FACTOR DEFICIENCIES)

Causes

Prothrombin (and factor VII) are formed in the liver by vitamin K, a fat-soluble vitamin contained in eggs and greens, but dietary deficiency is unknown, and normally some vitamin K is manufactured by bacteria in the intestine. Prothrombin deficiency is therefore due to:

(i) Failure of vitamin K absorption – obstructive jaundice, where there is a lack of bile salts, and, rarely, in malabsorption syndrome.

(ii) Liver dysfunction – cirrhosis, and in the newborn (haemorrhagic disease of the newborn).

(iii) Effects of drugs – the anticoagulant drugs phenindione and warfarin compete with vitamin K in the liver, blocking the formation of prothrombin – this is the basis of their therapeutic effect. Large doses of aspirin have a similar action. The breakdown of these drugs is increased by barbiturates and if the latter are added and subsequently withdrawn, rebound bleeding may occur.

Anticoagulant overdosage may present with haematuria, epistaxis or skin haemorrhages, and in all coagulation defects the blood is slow to clot after injury.

Haemophilia

Haemophilia is due to deficiency of factor VIII, antihaemophilic globulin. It is a sex-linked genetic disorder; thus it is transmitted by apparently normal females carrying the trait in one of their X chromosomes, and it affects only males.

Young boys are affected, but most now reach adult life. Patients bruise easily, and their blood does not clot well after injuries or dental extractions – there is a slow persistent ooze. Haemorrhage may occur into joints, causing pain and severe deformity if untreated.

Defibrination syndrome

This presents as continued severe bleeding and occurs in

concealed accidental haemorrhage in pregnancy (retro-placental bleeding), and following operations on the prostate or lungs. In both these situations there has been much bleeding and its continuation is due either to massive intravascular coagulation using up all the body's fibrinogen, or to excessive action of the fibrinolytic system attempting to dissolve the clots.

The diagnosis is established by finding a lack of fibrinogen in the blood, and there is failure of clot retraction when blood is allowed to clot in a test tube.

(3) POLYCYTHAEMIA

In polycythaemia there is an excess of circulating red cells, perhaps 7–8 $\times$ 10^{12}/l instead of the usual 5 $\times$ 10^{12}/l (7–8 million instead of 5 million/mm^3), a raised haematocrit (packed cell volume; normal 45%) and raised haemoglobin (over 120%).

Polycythaemia may be secondary to the anoxia of living at high altitudes, chronic lung disease (such as chronic bronchitis and emphysema) or cyanotic congenital heart disease.

Symptoms and signs

A feeling of fullness in the head, giddiness and fatigue.

'Ruddy' cyanosis.

A tendency to venous and arterial thrombosis and strokes.

A bleeding tendency.

Pruritus.

The spleen is enlarged in two-thirds of the cases.

(4) THE LEUKAEMIAS

Leukaemia is a neoplastic, malignant process affecting the white cells of the blood. Either the polymorph (the myeloid series), lymphocyte or monocyte series may be involved. There is an abnormal, progressive accumulation (hyperplasia) of cells in the haemopoietic tissues (bone marrow, lymph glands, spleen and liver) throughout the body and in chronic leukaemias increased circulating white blood cells.

Causes

In acute leukaemia the white cells fail to differentiate properly and build up in the bone marrow or lymph glands. In chronic leukaemia the accumulation may be due to a disturbance of the mechanism regulating the number that is normally produced.

The cause or causes are often obscure, but there is an increased incidence of leukaemia after exposure to X-rays or thermonuclear emissions as in the survivors of the atomic bomb explosions at Hiroshima and Nagasaki in 1945. A virus cause, an enzyme defect or a disorder of immunity are other possible causes.

Acute leukaemia

Acute leukaemia occurs especially in children and the cause is unknown. There is an accumulation of early cells ('blast' cells) in the marrow and lymph nodes. These cells fail to differentiate properly into their appropriate series, and crowd out other white cells, red cells and the platelets. The most common type in children is acute lymphatic (lymphoblastic) leukaemia, but in adults acute myelogenous leukaemia is equally common.

Symptoms and signs

A rapidly developing anaemia.

Haemorrhages (from platelet lack) from the gums and into the skin, bones and joints (causing severe pain in the latter) and internal organs, including the brain.

Fever, and susceptibility to infections.

Enlargement of lymph glands and spleen.

(Investigations include blood film and bone marrow examination.)

Chronic myeloid (granulocytic) leukaemia

The bone marrow and lymph glands are taken over by

abnormal cells usually found to contain an abnormal chromosome. There is a progressive accumulation of granulocytes (polymorphs) with an excess in the peripheral blood.

Symptoms and signs

Commonest in young adults.

Gradually increasing tiredness and weakness due to anaemia.

Enlargement of lymph glands, liver and spleen causing discomfort and 'dragging' sensation in the abdomen. Purpura and haemorrhages may occur.

Deposits in the skin and pruritus.

A raised metabolism with weight loss, sweats and raised blood uric acid causing gouty symptoms such as joint pains.

(The diagnosis is confirmed by finding a raised white blood cell count, sometimes over $100 \times 10^9/l$ (normal $4–9 \times 10^9/l$) in the peripheral blood, and by sternal or iliac marrow puncture.)

Chronic lymphatic leukaemia

The bone marrow is gradually infiltrated and eventually replaced by an accumulation of lymphocytes, also present in lymph nodes, spleen, liver and in the peripheral blood. In addition to progressive anaemia, the immunity function becomes defective and patients are prone to infection.

Symptoms and signs

Commonest in middle-aged and elderly men.

Tiredness, weakness.

Gland swellings and enlargement of the spleen.

May be remarkably benign in the elderly, being discovered sometimes at a blood count during investigations of pneumonia or other infection, or incidentally at a hospital attendance for another reason.

(The diagnosis is confirmed by a total white cell count of up to $100 \times 10^9/l$ ($100\,000/mm^3$), 90% of the cells being lymphocytes.)

Agranulocytosis

An absence or greatly decreased number (leukopenia) of white blood cells of the 'granular' series, the polymorphs, in the peripheral blood.

The cause is bone marrow depression, and the factors responsible are the same as in aplastic anaemia and thrombocytopenia, though some substances are more selective in destroying the white cells than the red cells or platelets.

The following drugs are the important causes:

phenylbutazone (butazolidin),
chloramphenicol,
anti-thyroid drugs such as carbimazole and methylthiouracil,
the cytotoxic drugs.

Symptoms and signs

The patient is prone to infection, and the first symptom is often a sore throat.

Marrow depression occurs over a longer period.

Fever and toxicity.

(5) DISORDERS OF THE SPLEEN AND LYMPH NODES

The spleen and lymph glands are the important filters in the defence system against foreign matter or organisms. The spleen is the filter for the circulating blood. The lymph glands are the filter for organisms arriving from the mucous membranes and skin via the lymphatics.

Functions

(a) Blood formation – the spleen's haemopoietic function can be increased if there is undue demand, or in marrow failure. The spleen has little reservoir function for red cells in man, but may store platelets.
(b) Blood destruction – the reticulo-endothelial cells remove red cells from circulation at the end of their 120-day life span.

(c) Defence against infection and participation in the immune response.

Causes of enlargement (splenomegaly)

(a) Infection – any severe, acute infection especially if there is bacterial invasion of the bloodstream as in typhoid fever or septicaemia ('septic' spleen):
  subacute bacterial endocarditis;
  chronic infections, especially tropical parasitic infections such as malaria and kala-azar (trypanosomiasis).

(b) Blood diseases:
  polycythaemia, myelosclerosis;
  the leukaemias;
  haemolytic anaemia, idiopathic thrombocytopenic purpura.

(c) Diseases of lymphoid tissue – Hodgkin's disease.

(d) Cirrhosis of the liver – causes portal venous obstruction.

Effects of splenomegaly

The spleen has to enlarge to about three times normal size before it becomes palpable. Enlargement is greatest in the tropical diseases, myelosclerosis and chronic myeloid leukaemia, where the size of the organ may cause discomfort. The spleen has an influence on bone marrow function, possibly hormonal, and 'hypersplenism' prevents release of cells from the marrow, causing anaemia, leukopenia or thrombocytopenia.

THE LYMPHATIC SYSTEM

Lymph is tissue fluid that enters the tiny lymphatic capillaries which join to drain it into the regional lymph nodes, where lymphocytes are added. The larger lymphatics terminate mainly in the thoracic duct, which enters the left subclavian vein at the root of the neck thus reaching the great veins near the heart. The lymphatic drainage of the small intestine is also an important route of fat absorption.

The lymphoid follicles in the lymph nodes produce the

lymphocytes concerned in humoral antibody and plasma cell formation.

Causes of lymph gland enlargement

(a) Infections: local, as from a septic fauces or sore throat: tuberculosis (and sarcoidosis) generalized, as in glandular fever (infectious mononucleosis).
(b) Metastatic: from spread of tumour cells along the lymphatics (for example axillary gland involvement from carcinoma of the breast).
(c) Primary malignant conditions of the haemopoietic system such as leukaemia, or of the lymphoreticular system – the reticuloses, such as Hodgkin's disease.

THE RETICULOSES

The cause or causes of the malignant reticuloses is unknown, but interest has been aroused by the finding of a rather similar tumour affecting the jaw and pharynx of children in tropical East Africa. This tumour was described by Burkitt and is called Burkitt's lymphoma. In some cases the cells contain a virus which may be transmitted by mosquitoes, and a similar virus may be found in glandular fever.

(a) Hodgkin's disease (lymphadenoma, malignant lymphoma)

Symptoms and signs

Commonest in young adults.

Swellings of the lymph glands, often first in the neck, the glands being rubbery but not tender.

Glands in the mediastinum (root of the lung) or abdomen may, however, be involved first, making diagnosis difficult – lymphatic blockage here may cause chylous ascites, or pressure on the veins may cause leg oedema.

Generalized glandular enlargement with enlarged spleen and liver.

Fever, weakness from anaemia.

Loss of weight and pruritus.

DIFFERENTIAL DIAGNOSIS OF ANAEMIA

	Onset	*Pre-existing conditions*
Anaemia – due to blood loss	may be acute or chronic	pallor, tachycardia, dyspnoea – may be post-traumatic or surgical; fatigue, angina
Anaemia – due to iron deficiency	chronic	peptic ulceration, salicylate usage, carcinoma, pregnancy, malnutrition; commonest in women
Anaemia – due to haemolysis	chronic, may be acute if induced	hereditary, haemoglobin or RBC abnormality; malaria drug usage, incompatible blood transfusion; chronic symptoms of anaemia
Pernicious anaemia	chronic, over years	middle-aged, elderly and predominantly female; anorexia, constipation, fatigue and chronic symptoms of anaemia

Associated findings	*Key laboratory findings*
hypotension if acute, shock; melaena, menorrhagia	routine RBC may not be abnormal in sudden loss, chronic loss gives reticulocytosis, low serum iron, Hb
menorrhagia, coeliac disease	low Hb, decreased RBCs, hypochromia, microcytosis, faecal occult blood positive; may have low serum folic acid as well as iron
Negroid or Mediterranean racial origin; jaundiced, spleno/hepatomegaly	low Hb, haemoglobin electrophoresis, may have porphyria, or sickle cell; G6PD deficiency; may have positive Coombs' test
glossitis, splenomegaly; peripheral neuritis	low Hb, macrocytic film; megaloblastic sternal marrow; low serum B_{12}

Investigations

Apart from anaemia and raised ESR, there are no specific findings in the peripheral blood. There may be infiltration of the bone marrow but the diagnosis of Hodgkin's disease is best confirmed by gland biopsy; lymphangiography defines its extent.

(b) Lymphosarcoma and reticulum cell sarcoma

These are malignant tumours of lymphoid tissue, involving lymphocytes and reticulum cells respectively. One of these cell types displaces all the others in lymph nodes, spleen, bone marrow or thymus gland. The process is much more rapid than in Hodgkin's disease and the cells spread into neighbouring tissues as well as spilling out via the lymphatics and bloodstream causing widespread dissemination of the growths. The condition may terminate as acute leukaemia.

Symptoms and signs

Similar to Hodgkin's disease, one group of nodes being first involved or the process presenting in several areas.

Mediastinal and retroperitoneal lymph nodes are frequently involved, causing discomfort, pressure symptoms and recurrent pleural or peritoneal effusions.

Lesions may start in the tonsils, stomach or other part of the alimentary tract, or present in the skin.

Malaise, fever, sweating and weight loss.

Anaemia occurs, sometimes haemolytic in type.

The diagnosis is confirmed by biopsy, which shows sheets of neoplastic cells of one cell type, different from the mixed cells in Hodgkin's disease tissue.

(c) Myelomatosis (multiple myeloma)

This condition occurs in the middle-aged and elderly, is commoner in men and is a malignant process usually arising in the bone marrow. Thus the marrow of flat bones such as the vertebrae and skull becomes infiltrated with plasma cells, called myeloma cells. There are single or multiple osteolytic (bone-destructive) lesions in the bony skeleton. The myeloma cells produce abnormal immunoglobulins, a product of which may appear as Bence Jones protein in the urine (see below). The cause is unknown.

Symptoms and signs

Bone pain and backache.

Fever, weight loss.

Anaemia and sometimes a bleeding tendency from thrombocytopenia.

Patients are prone to infection.

The weakened bones may fracture causing root pains such as a bilateral 'sciatica' if the vertebrae are involved.

The abnormal proteins may be deposited as amyloid tissue in nerves or organs including the tongue.

Deposits of protein in the renal tubules may cause renal failure.

Investigations

The ESR is raised – myelomatosis is a condition often associated with a very high ESR, 100 mm/h or more; such a finding may lead to the diagnosis in a patient with few symptoms. The abnormal proteins can be characterized by the procedure called paper strip electrophoresis, or by immunological methods.

On heating the urine, Bence Jones protein is detectable as a cloud around 70 °C, which disappears on boiling and reappears on cooling. When present, it is virtually diagnostic of myelomatosis.

X-rays show rarefaction or punched-out areas in the bones.

Chapter 14
The Psychological System

Psychological disorders, emotional and psychiatric, account for at least 20% of all medical consultations. Anxiety and depression form at least half of these, and the incidence in females is twice that of males. Hospitalization is (in order of frequency), for depression and suicide attempts, schizophrenia and other psychotic disorders, personality disorders, alcoholism, dementia and mental handicap. The most frequent cause of admission is for drug overdosage – now in some countries the single most frequent cause of all admissions to general hospitals. Suicide – self-poisoning – is the main cause of death in disorders of the psychological system.

Diagnosis of disorder will depend on symptoms, history, observation of the patient and examination of:

(A) disturbances of behaviour,
(B) psychological test performance,
(C) blood and urine tests (in drug abuse or overdosage).

Common symptoms of generalized disorder will be:

(1) psychological confusion: depression, anxiety, delusion, hallucination, coma;

(2) weight loss/excessive gain;
(3) multiple symptoms with suggestions of a physical hypochondria.

(A) DISTURBANCES OF BEHAVIOUR

Whilst history-taking or pursuing reported complaints of the psychologically disturbed patient, an irrationality and disconnected thought pattern can become obvious. Demeanour or dress, evidence of self-neglect, or inability to sit quietly describing symptoms soon reveal the disturbed personality. In doubt, relatives should always be interviewed as well as the patient.

(B) PSYCHOLOGICAL TESTS

Specific tests of intellectual/intelligence function can only be efficiently administered by those trained in their interpretation – simple tests of function with regard to asking name, date and for topical current information reveal inadequacies or confusional states.

(C) BLOOD AND URINE TESTS

In the overdosed or comatose patient, serum or urine levels for the commonly used or available drugs are essential for diagnosis and therapy management. It should always be recalled, however, that the suicidal patient may nevertheless have intercurrent physical disease and full health status assessment should be undertaken.

Common Disorders of the Psychological System

(1) MENTAL SUBNORMALITY (MENTAL RETARDATION)

Failure of normal brain development.

Causes include

chromosome abnormality, e.g. mongolism (Down's syndrome);

gene abnormality – phenylketonuria, an enzyme defect, excess amino acid (phenylalanine) damages brain;

damage to embryo – rubella (German measles) and toxoplasmosis in early pregnancy;

injury at birth;

post-natal – infections (e.g. meningitis); hypothyroidism if untreated (cretinism).

In many cases the cause is unknown.

The mentally subnormal may be assessed educationally according to Intelligence Quotient (IQ). Normal IQ is taken as 100. Those with an IQ over 80 may be educable normally, IQ 50–80 are subnormal and require special schooling, IQ under 50 are severely subnormal. Personality and emotional adjustment, family and social background influence management. The mentally handicapped may be better accepted in a rural community than in an industrial city.

(2) MENTAL ILLNESS

There are three main types of mental illness:
(a) due to an organic lesion;
(b) non-organic – psychiatric;
(c) personality disorders.

(a) DUE TO AN ORGANIC LESION

Where a known physical disease affects the brain, e.g. neurosyphilis, cerebral tumour, or arteriosclerosis, dementia, deterioration of intellect and memory, may result.

Toxic confusional states (delirium)

A toxic confusional state of delirium results from disordered function of the brain:

Causes

An organic cause – fever, infection, toxaemia, electrolyte depletion, hepatic failure (portal systemic encephalopathy), poisoning with alcohol or drugs, and, any condition causing cerebral anoxia;

A slight decrease in the oxygen supply to the brain cells is especially important where there is pre-existing brain damage or degeneration (as in dementia);

Thus respiratory infection or heart failure are common causes in the elderly – a toxic confusional state is reversible if the cause can be treated.

Symptoms and signs

There is clouding of consciousness;

Disorientation, confusion;

Restlessness;

Often accompanied by hallucinations (false perceptions);

The differentiation from an acute behaviour disturbance accompanying psychiatric illness such as schizophrenia or hysteria is not usually difficult, for in these there is no background of physical illness.

Dementia

Dementia is a deterioration of mental function following brain damage or disease – such damage is usually severe and extensive.

Causes

Dementia is usually a result of slowly progressive cerebral disease and is commonest in old age.

Senile dementia is seen especially in women and may be an ageing change – the brain undergoes shrinkage and plaques of degenerate tissue may be found at autopsy. Arteriosclerotic dementia also occurs in the elderly, especially in men, but can usually be differentiated by its association with previous strokes or other evidence of cerebral arterial disease, with or without hypertension: the deterioration of personality may not be so complete.

The pre-senile dementias are a group of conditions presenting in patients below the age of 60, e.g. Alzheimer's disease (probably an early form of senile dementia), Pick's disease, Huntington's chorea, and others – all relatively rare.

Neurosyphilis (GPI).

Cerebral tumour.

Chronic alcoholism.

Deficiency of thyroxine in myxoedema, or of vitamin B_{12} in pernicious anaemia are unusual causes.

Acute injury is a rare cause, but the repeated brain trauma sustained by boxers may lead to dementia.

Symptoms and signs

Impairment of intellect, associated with impairment of memory – the patient has a loss of memory for recent events but may be able to recall happenings of many years ago.

The memory disturbance causes disorientation in time and place.

A deterioration and coarsening of personality, and emotions may be shallow or disturbed.

Social behaviour disintegrates, personal appearance and hygiene are neglected.

The patient may become filthy in his toilet habits.

Conversation with the patient, enquiries as to name, address, age, and family ties, day of the month, current events, simple arithmetic (subtracting 7 from 100), giving numbers to remember – these usually suffice to confirm the diagnosis.

Dementia is usually a permanent state, but symptoms may be worsened by intercurrent infection or anoxia, especially in the elderly.

(b) NON-ORGANIC

(1) Anxiety and depressive states – a disturbance of the emotions or 'affect'. The patient retains his insight – he

realizes he is suffering from such a state. Anxiety neuroses include obsessive–compulsive states and phobias (irrational fears). Depressive illness is extremely common in all societies.

(2) Psychosis – a severe disorder in which the patient fails to realize he is mentally ill. Schizophrenia is the classical example, and the patient may be completely detached from reality.

(3) Psychosomatic and hysterical disorders – the patient has symptoms for which there is no physical basis.

Anxiety and depressive states

Anxiety and depression are extremely common. They may not be complained of, but will be admitted to, in many patients attending hospitals ostensibly with other complaints. They may be regarded as exaggerations of normal response to a stressful situation, grief and bereavement. While they may exist in 'pure' form as anxiety state and depressive state, they are commonly inseparable.

Symptoms and signs

A severe depressive state may present as anxiety.

Fears and feelings of unworthiness and guilt.

Complaints of sleeplessness and of feeling 'always tired'.

Depression may be classified as 'reactive' (i.e. reaction to an existing stressful situation such as financial trouble or a broken love affair), or 'endogenous' (in which the personality may basically be a depressive one and there may be a family history).

The reactive depressives have difficulty in getting off to sleep, whilst the endogenous depressives wake up in the small hours feeling extremely low in spirits and unable to get back to sleep.

Severe cases become extremely miserable and withdrawn, and unable to pursue their normal activities.

Concentration at book work becomes impossible.

Such patients may attempt suicide as the only relief from their misery.

The psychoses

A psychosis or psychotic state is a severe mental illness, in which the patient has no insight, and is often detached from reality.

The cause is unknown, but there may be a genetic predisposition and a biochemical abnormality in cerebral amine metabolism.

Symptoms and signs

Swings of mood from melancholia to acute excitement and violence amounting to mania. This is manic-depressive psychosis.

In mania, the patient appears uncontrollably excited with flights of idea, delusions (false beliefs) and hallucinations (false perceptions, the patient hearing or seeing things that are not there).

The term schizophrenia or schizophrenic psychosis is used to describe mental illness characterized by:

deterioration of emotional stability and personality;
disordered judgement; and
failure to act in accord with reality.

Schizophrenia presents in young people who, having been apparently normal, become withdrawn, decline to mix with others, and develop disorders of thought and of emotion. Abstract thinking is impaired, the thought process may suddenly become 'blocked' and the patient may believe that his thoughts are being influenced by outside sources – he may hear voices (auditory hallucinations), and there may be delusions of persecution, the paranoid state.

There is emotional flattening with swings from apathy to inappropriate laughter or outbursts of rage with aggression and destructiveness.

Mild cases often go unrecognized, the patient presenting himself repeatedly at hospital with many complaints, for which multiple investigations may have been carried out. The clue to such a state is the difficulty the doctor experiences in attempting to get a lucid history – after an hour's interview, he feels no further forward in the consultation.

(c) *PERSONALITY DISORDERS*

(1) Psychopathic disorder. A psychopath is a person who fails to conform to accepted social standards or conduct without being aware that he may be doing wrong. Psychopaths may be aggressive, creative, or socially inadequate.
(2) Alcoholism and drug dependence. Dependence exists when a person is compelled to take a drug for its psychic effects. Withdrawal may result in feelings so unpleasant that the habit is resumed.

It is becoming clear that many so-called mental disorders have a physical cause. Thus depression may be due to disturbed function of the emotional system connected with the hypothalamus, some schizophrenics have an abnormality of amine production, and an extra Y chromosome may be found in some criminal psychopaths. These considerations apart, physical illness may present as a mental illness such as depression. Again, the mental state of the patient affects his reaction to systemic disease.

Thus the division of mentally ill patients into a group to be kept apart in a special institution is no longer justified. The disturbed behaviour associated with mental disorders was often due to lack of understanding by relatives or doctors, leading to resentment and agitation in the patients who were quite unjustifiably confined behind locked doors. Some of the symptoms attributed to mental illness were in fact due to such institutionalization and social isolation. Modern psychiatric units are therefore part of the general hospital service.

Psychosomatic and hysterical disorders

Where there appears to be no physical basis for complaints, they are often labelled 'psychosomatic' or 'functional' or 'psychoneurotic'.

In hysteria the symptoms multiply and exhibitionism increases in front of an appropriate audience.

Hysteria is used in a different sense to describe a mental state in which part of normal consciousness is missing or 'detached'.

Symptoms and signs

There may be a hysterical paralysis of a limb, or the patient may fail to appreciate painful stimuli such as pin-prick, the sensory loss not conforming to a recognized pathological pattern.

Severe complaints may be described by a patient whose smiling appearance is incompatible with them.

Occasionally there may be memory loss or a 'fugue' in which the patient apparently does not know his or her identity and may be found wandering, by the police.

Hysterical fits, not of the pattern of true epilepsy, also occur.

The cause of such hysterical symptoms is uncertain, but personal gain may be the motive, albeit at subconscious level.

Anorexia nervosa

This is a condition found in the young. They stop eating, with marked loss of body weight, presenting an extreme emaciation in severe cases. The cause may be related to emotional disturbance or to an obsession that they are too fat and they proceed to put themselves on a starvation diet. They then develop a curious lack of insight into the fact that their physical appearance has become less, instead of more attractive. Amenorrhoea is usually present, but the secondary sexual characteristics such as pubic and axillary hair, are retained. Severe cases may go on to extreme weakness and death.

ALCOHOLISM

Acute alcoholic intoxication

The effects are well known – disturbance of balance, dysarthria, emotional and intellectual changes. Alcohol is a cerebral depressant, and while inhibitions may be released, judgement is impaired. There is a high association with road traffic accidents. Alcohol is also a gastric irritant, and a diuretic.

Chronic alcoholism

The alcoholic, or alcohol-dependent person, is one who has lost control of his drinking and cannot stop. He should be distinguished from the regular heavy drinker, who can still stop if advised to do so – signs of alcoholic poisoning such as peripheral neuropathy, cirrhosis, or alcoholic heart disease and failure are good reasons for this advice.

It is estimated that 1% of the population are alcoholics, but many conceal their addiction. They do not usually display signs of acute drunkenness, but their lives revolve around their need for alcohol. Alcoholism may follow excessive social drinking in those of previously good personality, or the habit may have followed a drinking bout after depression or stress, an escape from the 'cares of the world'. Some alcoholics have underlying psychotic disorders, many are psychopaths and the history often includes a broken home and family alcoholism.

Symptoms and signs

Morning drinking or solitary drinking may be the first signs.

The 'shakes' occurs on rising, following the withdrawal of alcohol during the period of sleep – there is tremor and irritability, and the subject reaches for another drink.

Gradually there is deterioration of personality and concentration at work, and all money is diverted to procuring alcohol – cheap wines (and sometimes methylated spirits) replacing the previous spirits.

Delirium tremens (DTs) is caused by intercurrent infection or sudden withdrawal of alcohol. Delirium is a state of clouding of consciousness, with restlessness and hallucinations – here they frequently take the form of small animals running over the body.

There is fear, confusion, and a tremor.

Encephalopathy is due to the vitamin B_1 deficiency common in the alcoholic, from poor diet.

There are haemorrhages at the base of the brain, causing confusion, paralysis of eye muscles with visual upset such as diplopia, nystagmus and ataxia.

This may proceed to loss of memory for recent events, and confabulation, the patient giving a fictitious account of his movements.

In the late stages of alcoholism there is progressive degeneration of cells in the cortex of the brain, with memory loss, intellectual deterioration and complete disintegration of standards of personal hygiene and behaviour.

DRUG DEPENDENCE (ADDICTION)

Dependence may be defined as a compulsion to take a drug on a continuous or period basis in order to experience its psychic effects and sometimes to avoid the discomfort of its absence. Thus withdrawal of some drugs of dependence results in symptoms such as agitation and anxiety – the brain has adapted to the drug and its absence may cause such symptoms, which may be related to a rebound excess activity of dream (REM) sleep. Tolerance to the drug, that is the need to take increasing doses to produce an effect, may or may not be present. Tolerance may be due to the production of increased enzymes by the liver, speeding destruction of the drug.

The introduction of opiates (morphine and heroin) has been followed by their misuse and dependence. Heroin mixed with cocaine (H and C) and injected intravenously ('mainlining') has euphoriant effects. These are powerful drugs of dependence and tolerance, so that subjects have to procure further supplies. Tight control has resulted in some improvement in heroin abuse in Britain, and addicts can only be supplied at special clinics. In the United States, however, heroin addiction remains a major problem.

Cannabis (marihuana, hashish, hemp, 'pot') is commonly smoked or eaten. It is said to remove inhibitions and improve the mood, giving a feeling of peace, but its effects are partly dependent on the subject's existing frame of mind and his social surroundings. Cannabis also causes dilatation of the conjunctival vessels. The smoke has a characteristic smell. Although there is no proof that its use has resulted in serious harm or dependence, those who smoke cannabis are at risk from their social associations with others who may use more dangerous drugs.

DIFFERENTIAL DIAGNOSIS OF ANXIETY AND DEPRESSION

	Onset	*Characteristics (subjective)*
Anxiety	acute or chronic	subjective feeling of apprehension, unease, tension, terror or panic; somatic complaints of headache, dyspnoea, hyperventilation, palpitation, dizziness, tremor, restlessness, fatigue, sweating; late night insomnia, anorexia
Depression	usually chronic, may be acute (e.g. grief)	pessimism, despair, sadness and irritability that is persistent; feelings of guilt, hopelessness, apathy; may be dramatic or delusional; may follow a swing from mania or hyperactivity in the young, may be more long-lasting in the elderly; obsessional and paranoid thoughts; anorexia, constipation, loss of libido, crying spells, early morning waking

Characteristics (objective)	*Laboratory investigations*
affects women more than men, onset in adolescence or early adulthood; episodes of abrupt onset; phobias and depressive reactions; frequent gastrointestinal disturbance; suicide rare	*Reassurance:* by complete blood count, urinalysis, thyroid function tests, GTT (if any evidence of hypoglycaemia); chest X-ray, exercise tolerance ECG, routine GIT investigation
affects elderly more than young, recurrent episodes become more chronic; may be agitated, careless of personal hygiene, memory impairment, delusions common, mental concentration deteriorates; suicide common	*To exclude organic cause:* complete blood count, urinalysis, serum electrolytes, thyroid function tests, chest X-ray, ECG, GIT investigation

LSD (lysergic acid diethylamide) and other derivatives produce hallucinations and may cause brain damage.

Almost any sedative or stimulant drug can be misused. Thus amphetamines cause stimulation but also psychotic episodes. Apart from such effects, intravenous use and sharing of syringes may result in sepsis and hepatitis. Amphetamines have little medical application, and curtailment of prescribing has resulted in less misuse. Thus drug-takers have turned to barbiturates and non-barbiturate hypnotics often mixed with alcohol, in their search for psychic effects.

Recent research suggests that disturbed beta-endorphin secretion in the brain may be related to drug and alcohol dependence.

(3) SELF-POISONING – ATTEMPTED SUICIDE

The vast majority of persons who take an overdose of drugs do so as an impulsive gesture, as a 'cry for help'. They will generally be admitted to hospital and they realize that their action affords an opportunity for their misery to be attended to. Only a small proportion intend to kill themselves and they make a planned attempt away from the public gaze, and, if foiled, try again. The term 'self-poisoning' is now therefore preferred to cover all cases with or without serious suicidal intent. Self-poisoning accounts for over 10% of acute admissions to British hospitals.

Corrosive acids and coal gas used to be the common methods, but the former is now regarded as unpleasant, and as natural gas contains no carbon monoxide, attempts with gas are ineffective. Car engine (petrol, not diesel) exhausts are, however, a source of carbon monoxide (and inadequate combustion or ventilation using any fuel can result in its production).

CARBON MONOXIDE POISONING

The gas fixes to haemoglobin, forming carboxyhaemoglobin and preventing oxygen carriage by the blood. Although carboxyhaemoglobin is pink, patients suffering from poisoning appear pink only if moribund. Earlier they are cyanosed and pale, confused or unconscious; breathing is maintained to a late stage.

ASPIRIN (SALICYLATE) POISONING

Acute aspirin poisoning does not initially cause unconsciousness in adults – even drowsiness is unusual though it does occur in children. If an adult patient with aspirin poisoning is unconscious, he is either at death's door, or another drug has been taken in addition.

Aspirin stimulates the respiratory centre causing rapid deep breathing. Though normal doses are antipyretic, overdosage causes metabolic stimulation, restlessness, pyrexia and sweating. There is tinnitus (noises in the ears). Gastric irritation causes vomiting and the patient becomes dehydrated. An initial respiratory alkalosis (due to over-breathing washing out CO_2) is followed by metabolic acidosis. There is potassium upset and hypokalaemia. Aspirin competes with vitamin K, resulting in lowered prothrombin level and bleeding tendency.

PARACETAMOL (ACETAMINOPHEN) POISONING

Paracetamol is contained in many proprietary analgesics and self-poisoning with the drug is now common – fatalities have occurred after ingestion of 10 g. Early symptoms include nausea, pallor and sweating but these may not be marked. Coma is not a feature unless other drugs have been ingested as well. Paracetamol overdosage damages the liver. An early assessment of the severity of the poisoning by measurement of blood paracetamol levels (a 4 h level over 200 mg/l being dangerous) is essential if treatment, which should be started within 10 h of ingestion, is to be effective.

Chapter 15

The Common Infections*

Almost half of any population at risk will be affected by one or other of the common infectious diseases in any one year. In the developed world, however, largely due to improvements in nutrition, the environment, and the use of antibiotics for the treatment of complications, specific infectious diseases – upper respiratory, chickenpox, measles, mumps, TB and hepatitis – account for less than 1% of deaths and less than 2% of hospital admissions.

Diagnosis of disorder will depend on symptoms, history, observation of the patient and examination of:

(A) blood tests, routine and for antibodies;
(B) exudates and mucus secretions for bacterial/viral identification;
(C) chest X-ray, where necessary.

Common symptoms of disorder will be:

(1) fever;
(2) anorexia, fatigue, malaise;

* See also chapter 5.

(3) rash;
(4) pain – headache, muscular, arthralgia or localized;
(5) nasal, skin, mucus discharge.

(A) BLOOD TESTS

The presence of specific disease detected by antibody formation depends on the time taken by the infected person to develop that response. Blood test initially demonstrating white cell changes brought about by a viraemia therefore may need to be repeated after a time interval to identify the specific antibody – rubella, infectious mononucleosis, influenza, brucellosis etc. – especially by means of a rising titre. Blood tests to identify the presence of the malaria parasite may only prove positive if taken at the time of the high fever. Diagnosis, therefore, by blood test is often only confirmatory of the suspicion engendered by the clinical signs.

(B) EXUDATE CULTURE

Viral growth from swabs of nasal discharge is not always readily available. Tubercle bacilli identification may require culture in living animal tissue and take time to achieve; gonococcal identification may be simply achieved by the immediate examination of a stained slide of urethral discharge. Thus a variation in the requirements of the laboratory for the identification of the specific disease may mean again that the diagnosis is confirmed, and not initially made by the bacteriology involved.

(C) CHEST X-RAY

This can be specific in cases of respiratory tuberculosis.

Common Infectious Diseases

(1) MEASLES

Measles is a virus infection usually affecting the young.

Symptoms and signs

Malaise, headache, fever.

Nasal discharge.

A rash involving the face and neck, spreading over the body.

White spots in the mouth near the molar teeth, Koplik's spots, may appear earlier, and are diagnostic.

Secondary bacterial invasion may cause middle-ear infections and pneumonia – while such complications are rare in the healthy, they are a common cause of death in measles outbreaks in underdeveloped countries.

(2) GERMAN MEASLES (RUBELLA)

Rubella is a virus infection.

Symptoms and signs

Mild malaise.

A pink rash about the neck, face, chest and abdomen.

Lymph gland swellings, especially the glands at the back of the neck. (The virus infects the developing embryo in the pregnant, resulting in congenital defects in the heart, brain, eye and ear.)

(3) SCARLET FEVER

Symptoms and signs

A scarlet rash, mainly affecting the trunk, occurring at the height of a haemolytic streptococcal sore throat.

The organism produces a toxin which affects the skin.

(4) WHOOPING COUGH

Symptoms and signs

The upper respiratory passages are affected, with appearances of a cough and cold.

The cough is followed by an inspiratory 'whoop' from laryngeal narrowing.

There may be vomiting.

(5) DIPHTHERIA

A bacterial infection of the throat causing pain.

Symptoms and signs

A 'dirty grey' membrane at the tonsillar region.

Cervical lymphadenopathy.

The production of a toxin affecting the heart and nervous system.

Any suspicion of this infection indicates the need for a throat swab to confirm diagnosis. Diphtheria may occur as an infection of the larynx alone and should be borne in mind in cases of hoarseness with systemic upset.

(6) CHICKENPOX (VARICELLA)

The virus is the same as that causing herpes zoster (shingles) in adults. Susceptible children may develop chickenpox following contact with cases of shingles, but the reverse is unusual.

Symptoms and signs

Mild febrile disease with a rash that comes in crops.

Stages of red spots, then fluid-containing vesicles, pustules – with much itching – and scabs which fall off without leaving a scar.

The neck, shoulders and trunk are especially affected.

(7) SMALLPOX (VARIOLA)

One of the recent triumphs of preventive medicine is the virtual elimination of smallpox throughout the world, through the successful campaign of the World Health Organization.

Smallpox was a highly infectious and contagious disease

with serious epidemics throughout the centuries causing death and disfigurement. Now, however, the last report of smallpox resulting from person-to-person transmission was in Somalia in 1977, and 1978 would have been a clear year had two cases of infection not occurred from a laboratory in Birmingham (UK). Since the risks of vaccination now outweigh the risks of acquiring the infection, smallpox vaccination is no longer compulsory and the number of countries requesting an International Certificate of Vaccination is gradually declining.

Symptoms and signs

Fever.

Toxaemia and a characteristic rash of spots.

Vesicles and pustules (which swarm with the virus), affecting the face and trunk.

These might become haemorrhagic leaving scarring. The victim may die of complicating pneumonia or cardiac failure.

The diagnosis is confirmed by electronmicroscopy recognition of the virus from the skin lesions.

(8) MUMPS (PAROTITIS)

Mumps is a virus infection of the parotid glands at the angle of the jaw, and infection is transmitted in the saliva. It is a relatively trivial infection in children, and epidemics tend to occur in schools – incubation period is up to 3 weeks.

Symptoms and signs

Fever.

Difficulty in opening the mouth and chewing, with parotid gland swelling.

The virus may invade the nervous system causing a form of meningitis.

Complications include orchitis (inflammation of the testis, usually unilateral) and pancreatitis.

(9) INFLUENZA

Influenza is a virus infection, mainly affecting the upper respiratory tract.

Symptoms and signs

Cough, sneezing and sore throat.

Fever, headache and limb pains.

Often prostration out of proportion to the respiratory signs.

It is a short, sharp illness (lasting 4–5 days), but in those with lung disease there is risk of secondary, often staphylococcal pneumonia.

(10) INFECTIOUS MONONUCLEOSIS (GLANDULAR FEVER)

This is an acute infection from EB (Epstein–Barr) virus (which is also found in Burkitt's lymphoma, a glandular swelling in East African children). Outbreaks of infectious mononucleosis tend to occur in young people living communally.

Symptoms and signs

Sore red throat, often with tonsillar exudate is common, and distinguishable from streptococcal throat only by the negative throat swab in glandular fever.

Lymph gland swelling, especially in the neck.

The spleen may be palpable.

Liver involvement may cause jaundice.

Diagnosis is confirmed by blood film, which shows 'mononuclear' cells – altered lymphocytes, and a positive 'Paul Bunnell' or 'Monospot' test on the serum.

(11) TUBERCULOSIS

Tuberculosis is due to infection with the tubercle bacillus, *Mycobacterium tuberculosis*, termed an 'acid-fast' bacillus as it resists the decolorizing effect of acid used to stain the organism for identification under the microscope. It can be cultured on special media, or if the organisms are scanty, guinea-pig inoculation (the animal manifesting the infection after 6 weeks) may establish their presence.

Mode of infection is by inhalation of droplets of infected sputum into the lungs. A primary focus occurs in the lung tissue, with involvement of lymph glands near the root of the lung. When tuberculosis was common, this occurred in most young people; usually the infection would heal and the subject become immune to further infection. If resistance was low, dissemination throughout the body – miliary tuberculosis – could occur. This might result in tuberculous meningitis, previously fatal, or chronic infection in bones and kidneys.

Alternatively, the primary infection might become reactivated, following a lowered resistance or reinfection, in adult life, leading to tuberculous pneumonia or to chronic fibrocaseous tuberculosis of the lungs, with much destruction cavity formation, and the expectoration of purulent sputum containing the tubercle bacilli.

Undiagnosed tuberculosis of this type is the present source of infection.

Symptoms and signs

Cough, sputum, and weight-loss are late signs.

Early recognition depends on chest X-ray. (X-ray is mandatory in all undiagnosed fevers, even if chest symptoms are minimal.)

TB meningitis may present as headache and mild neck stiffness, lumbar puncture showing increased cells, decreased sugar and the TB bacillus in the spinal fluid.

Diagnosis is confirmed by finding the organism on direct staining, culture, or guinea-pig inoculation of sputum, cerebrospinal fluid, or urine.

(12) BRUCELLOSIS (UNDULANT FEVER)

Cause

Brucella abortus – a small bacterium named after Bruce (who discovered a similar organism causing Malta fever), and the tendency of infected cattle to abort their young. Veterinary surgeons, farmers, and those who drink the milk of infected animals may contract the disease, which has been eradicated in some progressive farming countries. Pasteurization is a measure to render existing milk supplies safe.

Symptoms and signs

Vague ill-health.

Aches and pains.

Fever and night-sweats.

Severe cases may have inflammation of spinal and other joints. The infection may be acute, or last for months, and should be considered in any vague pyrexia.

Diagnosis may be confirmed by positive tests for antibodies in the blood (e.g. agglutination test) and Brucellin skin test.

(13) VENEREAL DISEASE

The venereal diseases are acquired from infected persons at sexual intercourse, and they have increased in recent years. The defined venereal diseases are gonorrhoea, syphilis, and soft chancre, but other sexually transmitted diseases include non-specific urethritis and some cases of vaginitis from the trichomonas parasite.

Gonorrhoea

Cause

The gonococcus, a Gram-negative bacterium seen on microscopy, or by culture.

Symptoms and signs

Purulent urethral discharge in males, with dysuria.

Females may have vaginal and urethral discharge, and infection may involve the ovarian tubes causing sterility, but many female carriers are symptom-free.

Occasionally there is an acute gonococcal arthritis.

The eyes of newborn babies may be infected from contact with vaginal secretions at birth.

Syphilis

Cause

A bacterium of spirochaete (corkscrew-like) group called *Treponema pallidum*. Like the gonoccocus, the organism fails to survive outside the body and is acquired only by contact with an infected lesion, usually at intercourse. There is a delay of up to a month, during which the treponemes have spread throughout the body, before signs appear.

Symptoms and signs

Primary stage
A syphilitic sore or chancre on the penis, or the vulva.

Secondary stage
Skin rashes and generalized lymph gland enlargement with involvement of blood vessels and nervous system – meningovascular syphilis.

Tertiary stage (after a latent period of up to 15 years)
Heart involvement – syphilitic inflammation of the root of the aorta causing aortic valve incompetence, and dilatation (aneurysm) of aorta.

Central nervous system
  tabes dorsalis (ataxia, shooting pains);
  general paralysis of the insane (dementia).

Gumma – abscess-like swelling affecting any organ.

Congenital syphilis occurs from infection in the uterus, the baby being stillborn or with deformities of brain, teeth and bones.

Diagnosis

The spirochaete may be seen under the microscope (dark-ground illumination) in smears from early lesions. Later

DIFFERENTIAL DIAGNOSIS OF COMMON INFECTIONS

	Age of onset	*Distinguishing features*
Measles	children	follows apparent URTI, Koplik's spots in mouth, confluent erythematous rash
Rubella	children/ young adults	cervical/occipital lympadenopathy, confluent rapidly (48 h) clearing rash
Scarlet fever	children	'scarlet' rash mainly on trunk, septic throat
Whooping cough	children	characteristic inspiratory whoop with paroxysms of coughing
Diphtheria	children/non-immune adults	severely sore throat, grey membrane, severe toxaemia and dysphagia, stridor
Chickenpox	children/non-immune adults	separate discrete vesicular spots, arising in crops, central in distribution
Smallpox	any age	vesicles and pustules, some haemorrhagic centripetal in distribution
Mumps	children/ young adults	swollen salivary glands and moon face of bilateral parotitis, accompanying orchitis sometimes and abdominal pains
Influenza	any age	prostration and pyrexia disproportionate to the obvious upper respiratory infection; limb aches and severe headache
Mononucleosis	children/ young adults	sore throat and tonsillar exudate with slough, generalized lymphadenopathy, splenomegaly and jaundice sometimes
Tuberculosis	any age	respiratory – chronic productive cough with, in severe cases, haemoptysis
Brucellosis	any age	vague, recurrent symptoms including night sweats and generalized lassitude
Malaria	any age/ traveller in exposure area	rigors and severe fever with a pattern of progressive temperature rise and sweats

Key laboratory findings
viral culture possible – diagnosis made by rash
serum antibodies rise
throat swab grows streptococcus
culture of sputum, nasal and throat swabs; cough diagnostic
throat swab, serum antibodies (skin test in immune)
diagnosis by rash – viral culture of vesicle
viral culture of vesicle
salivary swab culture – diagnosis by appearance; serum antibody titre
nasal viral culture; serum antibodies
blood film diagnostic with excess mononuclear cells; antibodies demonstrable; positive Paul–Bunnell and 'Monospot' test
X-ray diagnostic; sputum culture of acid-fast bacilli and guinea-pig inoculation; Mantoux skin test
antibody titre rise; Brucellin skin test
parasites seen in fresh stained blood film

diagnosis depends on blood antibody tests, such as the VDRL (Reference Laboratory), WR (Wasserman reaction) and treponemal fluorescent antibody and immobilization tests. Cerebrospinal fluid tests are also necessary in secondary and tertiary stages.

Non-specific urethritis

This presents as a urethral discharge, from which gonococci are absent, up to 2 months after sexual intercourse. Some cases are due to infection with *Chlamydia* (an organism associated with the eye disease trachoma in the tropics) but in others the organism is unknown. There may be associated conjunctivitis (inflammation of the outer covering of the eye) and arthritis (lumbar spine and joints of the feet being involved), the condition called Reiter's syndrome.

(14) MALARIA

Incidence and cause

Malaria is a common tropical disease, and should be remembered as a cause of fever in travellers from such parts. It is due to infection with a parasite, of which there are several types, which undergoes part of its life-cycle in certain mosquitoes which bite man. The parasite passes from the salivary glands of the mosquito to the bloodstream of man, invading the liver and the red blood cells, destruction of the latter coinciding with the bouts of fever characteristic of the infection. Native populations develop a natural immunity, and those carrying the 'sickle cell' trait (from an abnormal haemoglobin) are protected against severe malaria.

Symptoms and signs

There is a 'cold stage' with shivers and rigors, followed by high fever with headache and malaise.

The temperature later subsides, with marked sweating.

The spleen may be palpable.

Diagnosis

Confirmed by finding the parasites in blood films. In severe cases there may be drowsiness, fits and coma – cerebral malaria, and sometimes hypotension and collapse, with severe haemolysis (breakdown of red cells) and darkly pigmented urine (blackwater fever).

(15) TETANUS

Cause

A bacillus, *Clostridium tetani*, which inhabits the intestine of horses and sheep, forming spores found in manure, soil and dust. The bacillus grows in the absence of oxygen in deep puncture wounds and injuries – but these may be trivial ones, or apparently healed. The bacilli produce a toxin which travels up the peripheral nerves to the central nervous system.

Symptoms and signs

Discomfort and stiffness at the wound, followed by spasm of the jaw muscles (hence the name lockjaw) within a few days, or a few weeks, the latter giving a better prognosis.

This is followed by painful general spasms of muscle, precipitated by stimuli such as movement or even a loud noise.

These spasms may cause ultimate exhaustion and death.

Index